Health Care and the Changing Economic Environment

Health Care and the Changing Economic Environment

Alan L. Sorkin
University of Maryland

Lexington Books
D.C. Heath and Company/Lexington, Massachusetts/Toronto

Library of Congress Cataloging in Publication Data

Sorkin, Alan. L.
    Health care and the changing economic environment.

    Includes index.
    1. Medical economics—United States. 2. Medicare. 3. Medicaid. I. Title. [DNLM:
1. Delivery of Health Care—economics—United States. 2. Economics, Medical—trends—
United States. W 74 S714hb]
RA410.53.S67   1986   338.4′ 33621′ 0973   84-47976
ISBN 0-669-09016-6 (alk. paper)

Second printing, January 1987
Published simultaneously in Canada
Printed in the United States of America
International Standard Book Number: 0-669-09016-6
Library of Congress Catalog Card Number: 84-47976

The paper used in this publication meets the minimum requirements of American National
Standard for Information Sciences—Permanence of Paper for Printed Library Materials,
ANSI Z39.48-1984.

In memory of my mother
Sally E. Sorkin
1911–1985

Contents

Tables

Preface and Acknowledgments

The health care industry has always been an industry of dynamic change. New types of health manpower were created in response to the physician shortage of the 1960s. Many drugs and diagnostic procedures in use today have been developed within the past five years. New surgical interventions such as heart (both real and artificial) and liver transplants give patients the opportunity for prolonged life.

However, the medical care industry is presently being affected by two phenomena which are unique to the 1980s. These forces have elements that are independent of each other, but have aspects that are interdependent as well.

The first phenomenon is related to the cutbacks in federal health care programs which are an outgrowth of rising federal budget deficits during a period when the executive branch has been dominated by a conservative political philosophy. These reductions in federal health care spending threaten access to health care by the poor, elderly, and some categories of veterans.

The second major factor currently affecting the health care industry is the increase in competition between various providers. This competition between hospitals, health maintenance organizations, and walk-in clinics reflects the growing emphasis by various third-party payers on cost containment. In addition, the rapid increase in the supply of physicians is increasing competition between doctors and causing pressure for reductions in training programs for physician assistants and nurse practitioners.

The book will focus on the ways in which the health care industry is adapting to the changing economic environment. Whenever possible, the material is presented in a nontechnical manner in order to be readily understood by those without extensive formal training in either health economics or health administration.

The first draft of the manuscript was typed by Iris Batchellor. Subsequent drafts were typed by Peggy Bremer. Both of them did an excellent job in preparing the manuscript for publication.

Bruce Katz read the manuscript and made a number of helpful comments. However, the author alone is responsible for any errors of fact or interpretation. The manuscript was edited by Bruce Sylvester, and the index was prepared by Sallie Steele.

1
Introduction

The past fifteen years have witnessed a rapid improvement in the health status of the American population. Significant reductions in mortality from ten of the fifteen leading causes of death have occurred. Moreover, infant and maternal deaths have fallen greatly, particularly among blacks and American Indians. From 1968 to 1980, life expectancy increased by four years.[1]

Although not all of these improvements in health status are solely attributable to more or better medical care, these gains occurred simultaneously with the greatest public and private effort to improve health care in the history of the United States. These gains also happened during a time of focused effort to improve access to medical services for the elderly and some categories of low-income persons.

While the health care industry grew rapidly in the 1960s and 1970s, with little attempt to limit expenditures, the 1980s have brought an emphasis on cost-containment measures. Moreover, since health expenditures now account for more than a tenth of gross national product (GNP), there is increased concern regarding the efficiency and effectiveness of the services provided by the medical care industry.

Some of this concern is associated with a changing economic environment. The recent decade has been one of below-average economic growth, slow productivity gains, and rapid inflation. Limited income gains have contributed to massive federal budget deficits as tax revenues have fallen further and further behind government expenditures. The budget deficit was $79 billion in 1981, $128 billion in 1982,[2] and over $200 billion in 1983, 1984, and 1985. Partly because of these record-breaking peacetime deficits, the government has responded by cutting social programs including health activities such as Medicare, Medicaid, and veterans' health programs. Moreover, the president is proposing further budget cuts of $52.1 billion in 1986, and up to $100 billion by 1988.[3]

The president has proposed an additional $5 billion reduction in the federal contribution to the Medicaid program from 1986 to 1988, and a cut nearly four times that large in the Medicare program over the same time period. Funding for veterans' health care would also decline. Although there are differences between the major political parties concerning which sectors should absorb the brunt of these budget reductions, it is likely that health care programs would absorb some cuts even if the House and Senate were both under the control of the Democratic party.

One implication of these cutbacks (if they are sustained by Congress) is that the gains which have occurred in health care access may be imperiled. The share of the nation's low-income population covered by Medicaid has fallen from 65 percent in 1976 to 52 percent in 1984.[4] If the president's proposed Medicaid reduction actually occurs, further reduction in program participation among the poor can be expected. Moreover, Medicare budget reductions will result in rising premiums and deductibles, meaning that the elderly will be expected to pay a rising proportion of their health care costs.

Employers as well as the government are trying to restrict health care spending. The percentage of employers requiring employees to pay deductibles for inpatient hospital care has gone from 30 percent in 1982 to 63 percent in 1984.[5] Moreover, in order to limit cost increases, employers are switching from conventional health insurance for their employees to health maintenance organizations (HMOs) or preferred provider organizations (PPOs).

Along with the emphasis on cost containment, the health care industry is becoming more competitive. Walk-in clinics, ambulatory surgery centers, free-standing emergency centers, and alternative birth centers are all examples of relatively new types of health care organizations which are competing with hospitals for patients. In response, hospitals have opened their own ambulatory surgery centers, allocated space for luxurious birthing rooms, and established HMOs and satellite clinics. They have also begun to advertise extensively.

Many of these newer types of health care organizations are privately owned by either physician–entrepreneurs or groups of investors. In addition, the fastest growing segment of the hospital industry is the proprietary hospital chain. Not only do these chains operate their own facilities on a for-profit basis, but they are managing an increased proportion of the nonprofit hospitals. Recently these corporate chains have even begun acquiring or managing teaching hospitals and urban hospital centers. There is concern that the growing for-profit hospital sector may neglect the poor nonpaying patient and reduce the emphasis on medical research. However, there is some evidence that corporate hospital chains are able to deliver services at lower cost than nonprofit hospitals.

Not only is there increased competition among health care facilities, but there is growing competition among medical personnel. Because of the growing supply of health manpower, physicians and other health care providers face increased competition for patients. This may result in certain positive social benefits. More physicians may be willing to attend to the medical needs of Medicaid and other low-income patients. Others may be willing to move to underserved areas such as the rural South or Southwest, and some may adjust their office hours to reflect a greater convenience to their patients.

One likely result of the growing supply of physicians is much greater scrutiny of the process of awarding medical licenses. This may cause reductions in the number of foreign medical graduates who are permitted to practice in this country, as well as increased efforts to prevent cheating on the major licensing examinations such as the National Board Exam.

Plan of This Book

This book will consider the impact of the changing economic environment on the nation's health care system. In addition, the effect of increased competition and the growth of the for-profit segment of the health care industry will be explored.

Chapter 2 presents statistical information on the long-term rise in health care expenditures. It discusses some of the more important reasons for this rapid increase in expenditures such as health sector inflation; the role of third-party payers, namely insurance companies and government, in stimulating demand; and the costs associated with the increased tendency of patients to file malpractice suits.

Chapter 3 traces the shift in the quantity of health manpower from shortage to probable surplus. The implications of increased competition among providers are discussed in some detail.

Chapter 4 is a multidimensional consideration of the Medicare program. This program will likely face a major financing crisis by the early 1990s. Various options which will postpone or avert this crisis are discussed. The expected impacts of the prospective payment system for hospitalized Medicare patients are analyzed.

Chapter 5 focuses on various aspects of hospital economics. The impact of health sector inflation has been greatest in the hospital industry, and hospitals have strongly felt the impact of the increasingly competitive health care environment. Walk-in clinics and ambulatory surgery centers have caused a significant drop in inpatient occupancy rates and outpatient visits. Both state agencies and the federal government have been increasingly active in regulating the hospital industry, particularly in the area of cost containment. However, if reimbursement controls are pushed too aggressively, hospitals may suffer chronic deficits, for example, or be forced to reduce the quality of care.

Chapter 6 examines the Medicaid program. Like Medicare, the Medicaid program has been a target of administration cutbacks. Many physicians do not accept Medicaid patients because of relatively low reimbursement levels.

Further cutbacks may make it more difficult for Medicaid-eligible persons to obtain care. In addition, there is evidence that patients dropped from the Medicaid program suffer a relative decline in health status compared to those remaining in the program.

Chapter 7 considers the economic implications of health maintenance organizations. HMOs have had a smaller impact on the health service industry than their advocates anticipated. One reason for this lack of impact is the reluctance of HMOs to compete vigorously with each other or with other health care organizations.

The final chapter discusses some of the newer approaches to health care delivery. Many of these new kinds of organizations deliver care for far less money than do hospitals. Most of these clinics and centers are privately owned. This is one important dimension of the increasing privatization of the health care industry. There is a recent tendency toward licensing or accrediting these relatively new forms of health care. It is likely that increasing pressure for these forms of quality control will come from third-party payers in an effort to protect the consumer and encourage the provision of cost-effective medical care.

This book describes a health system in transition. The role of the private (for-profit) sector in the provision of medical care is clearly increasing. This trend toward privitization has a number of consequences, which are discussed throughout the book.

Notes

1. David Rogers and Robert Blendon, "Checking for Symptoms of Declining Health Care," *Wall Street Journal,* September 12, 1984, p. A-1.

2. Congressional Budget Office, *The Economic and Budget Outlook: An Update* (Washington, D.C.: U.S. Government Printing Office, 1983), pp. 2–7.

3. Helen Dewar, "Reagan, Senators Agree on Package to Trim Deficit," *The Washington Post,* April 24, 1985, p. A-1.

4. Rogers and Blendon, op. cit.

5. Ibid.

2
Health Care Expenditures

E
xpenditures on health services for medical care in the United States in 1983 reached $355.4 billion, a 10.2 percent increase from 1982 levels and roughly 11 percent of the GNP. This amounted to $1,459 per person in 1983, the highest national per capita health expenditure in the world, and approximately 100 times the $10 to $15 per capita expenditure on health services in developing countries. By comparison, during 1975, U.S. health care expenditures were $132.7 billion, which represented 8.4 percent of the GNP, while in 1950, expenditures were only 4.6 percent of the GNP. Thus, in thirty-three years, health care expenditures as a fraction of the GNP have more than doubled in the United States.[1] (See table 2–1.)

Among the factors accounting for the rapid growth in medical expenditures are a major increase in the demand for health services, recently augmented by a large rise in government financing; changing methods of prepaying for health care, including continuous growth of insurance; the rapid and sustained increase in health care prices; and the rising level of malpractice claims.

A recent study projects the level of health care expenditures at $690 billion in 1990, and $1.9 trillion by the year 2000. Per capita expenditures are projected to rise to $2,760 in 1990, and $6,700 by the year 2000. This projection to some extent reflects the recent historical pattern in which total health expenditures have approximately doubled every six years. The study estimates that total health expenditures will be 12 percent of the GNP in 1990 and 14 percent in 2000.[2] If this latter figure is correct, it implies a doubling of the proportion of GNP devoted to health services from 1970 to 2000.

Why has the proportion of output devoted to health services increased so rapidly? First, it is generally accepted that, as an economy matures, consumers spend an increasing proportion of income on services, including medical care. Second, as an economy undergoes the process of development, industries with below average productivity growth will experience more rapid price inflation than industries with above average productivity gains.[3] Health care, despite recent advances in technology, is still quite labor intensive, and has experienced below average productivity growth. Third, rapid

Table 2-1
Expenditures for Health and Medical Care in the United States, Selected Years, 1929–1983
(billions of dollars)

Type of Expenditure	1929	1940	1950	1960	1970	1975	1980	1982	1983
Total (dollars)	3.60	4.00	12.70	26.90	68.00	132.70	247.20	322.40	355.40
Private expenditures	3.11	3.02	9.86	19.46	42.86	75.81	143.00	185.60	206.60
Health and medical services[a]	3.01	2.99	9.64	18.94	40.69	72.74	139.00	179.90	199.70
Medical facilities construction	.10	.03	.22	.52	2.17	3.07	4.00	5.70	6.90
Public expenditures	.48	.78	3.07	6.40	25.23	56.31	104.20	136.80	148.80
Health and medical services	.37	.66	2.47	5.35	22.58	51.34	96.90	128.70	140.40
Medical research	—	.03	.07	.47	1.65	2.98	5.10	5.60	5.80
Medical facilities construction	.10	.09	.52	.58	1.00	1.99	2.20	2.50	2.60
Total expenditures as a percentage of GNP	3.60	4.00	4.60	5.20	7.10	8.60	9.40	10.50	10.80
Public expenditures as a percentage of total expenditures	13.33	19.50	24.17	23.79	37.10	42.43	42.15	42.43	41.87
Personal care expenditures	3.17	3.50	10.40	22.73	59.13	116.80	217.90	286.90	313.30
Private expenditures	2.89	2.98	8.30	17.80	38.58	70.60	131.50	171.20	188.80
Public expenditures	.28	.52	2.10	4.93	20.55	46.20	86.40	115.70	124.50
Percentage from private expenditures	91.10	85.10	79.80	78.30	65.20	60.40	60.40	59.70	58.10
Direct payments	88.50	82.80	68.30	55.50	39.40	32.40	31.40	27.20	
Insurance benefits	—	—	8.50	20.70	24.40	26.70	26.70	26.70	31.90
Percentage from public expenditures	8.90	14.90	20.20	34.80	39.60	40.10	39.70	40.30	41.90

Source: Alfred Skolnik and Sophie Dales, "Social Welfare Expenditures, 1972–1973," *Social Security Bulletin* 37, no. 1 (January 1974):13; Robert Gibson, "National Health Expenditures, 1979," *Health Care Financing Review*, (Summer 1980):17–18, 23; Health Care Financing Administration, Office of Research, Demonstrations, and Statistics, "Health Care Financing Trends" (Summer 1981):2; U.S. Department of Health and Human Health Services, *Health: United States, 1981*, DHHS Publication No. (PHS) 82-1232 (Washington, D.C.: U.S. Public Health Service, 1982), pp. 263–64, 268; Robert Gibson, Daniel Waldo, and Katherine Levit, "National Health Expenditures, 1982," *Health Care Financing Review* 5, no. 1 (Fall 1983):6, 8; Robert Gibson, Katherine Levit, Helen Lazenby, and Daniel Waldo, "National Health Expenditures, 1983," *Health Care Financing Review* 6, no. 2 (Winter 1984):3, 7–8.

[a]Includes medical research.

advances in, and diffusion of medical technology have expanded the treatment of a wide variety of diseases and other medical conditions. This has resulted in greater consumption of health care per capita as consumers and health care providers utilize the most modern facilities and equipment available. Fourth, the population of the United States is aging. While each age group is healthier than its counterparts of previous decades, one consequence of an aging population is rising consumption of health services: older people require more hospital and nursing home care than do younger people.

These sources of growth in health care expenditures reflect long-term changes of a gradual nature. A fifth cause of increases in the share of GNP allocated to health care reflects the way in which that care is financed. Two factors are important in this regard: third-party reimbursement and government subsidies of health care spending. More than in any other market for consumer goods and services, third parties, rather than consumers themselves, pay for the utilization of health services. The extent of third-party reimbursement for health care ranges from 88 percent of hospital expenditures to 22 percent of spending for consumer medical durables and nondurables including drugs and eyeglasses.[4]

Third-party reimbursement leads to greater consumption of health care for two reasons. First, when a third party pays for a service, the consumer is often unaware of the actual cost of the service. Because the perceived price is below the actual price, consumers use more health care services than they would if they had to pay the full cost themselves. Second, until recently, most third-party reimbursement has been cost-based or retrospective in nature. When the insurer paid a large proportion of costs, regardless of the amount of those costs, there was little incentive for consumers or providers of care to be cost conscious. Retrospective financing reflected the original intent of health insurance, which was to guarantee access to health care whatever the level of total expenditures. However, with the rapid increase in health care expenditures, the cost-based aspect of third-party reimbursement has generated increasing pressure for reform.

Another important factor affecting the financing of health care is the tax treatment of both health insurance premiums and out-of-pocket payments for health care. Under present law, employer contributions for health insurance policies are excluded from employees' taxable income and from earnings subject to payroll taxes. In addition, up to $150 of an employee's share of health insurance premiums could be deducted directly from taxable income until 1982; and the remainder of those premiums, along with other consumer medical expenses, were tax deductible if they exceeded 3 percent of adjusted gross income (5 percent after 1982). The tax treatment of premiums alone cost the federal government $26 billion in foregone revenue in fiscal year 1983.[5] The tax-exempt status of health insurance premiums encourages employees to substitute more comprehensive insurance coverage for higher money wages. Many consumers view such expanded insurance coverage as a costless benefit, and tend to overconsume health care services, even though such overconsumption raises the price of health insurance in the long run. Tax treatment of health care spending and the extent of third-party coverage of health care are fundamental causes of rising health expenditures.

Government response to increasing health care expenditures and rapidly growing federal budget deficits has been to constrain expenditures for federal programs such as Medicare and Medicaid. Thus, states have been authorized to limit the services and populations covered by Medicaid and to institute copayments for Medicaid services. (See chapter 6.) California has recently instituted a system in which hospitals bid for the right to admit Medicaid patients. The deductible and coinsurance rates charged for various services under the Medicare program have been increased. (See chapter 5.) A major break from retrospective reimbursement was begun under Medicare with the adoption of prospective reimbursement for hospitals, a policy to take effect gradually between fiscal years 1984 and 1986. Patients are classified upon diagnosis into one of several hundred diagnosis-related groups (DRGs). Thus, a hospital knows at the time of admission how much Medicare will pay for treatment of the patient. This knowledge is expected to make providers of care become more cost conscious. One other cost measure is a freeze of Medicare physician fee schedules. It is hoped that these and other policies will result in greater recognition of the actual cost of care, both by consumers of that care and by its providers, and that growth of health care expenditures will be retarded.

Rising health expenditures also reflect the fact that some services once provided free of charge by household members are now provided by health professionals. This factor contributes to growth in the health sector and is of particular importance for one of the fastest growing services, long-term care. The increasing proportion of females sixteen years of age and over who are in the labor force contributes to the change in the way these services are provided. This proportion increased from 39 percent in 1965 to 57 percent in 1984, resulting in a smaller number of persons available for productive, nonpaying work in the household. Because more women are working, the opportunity cost of providing unpaid personal care services for relatives and friends has sharply increased. In addition, the size of the average household fell from 3.3 persons in 1965 to 2.7 in 1981,[6] a decline of 18 percent. As average household size decreases due to social, economic, and demographic forces, there are fewer household members to provide personal care.

Thus, as more women join the labor force and as the average household size decreases, some long-term health care activities have been pushed out of the household and into the health sector market. It is likely that increased third-party payments for coverage of health services have intensified this trend.

It is possible that providers induce some of the demand for their services. The patient's dependence upon the physician for technical decisions and the existence of third-party payments may result in higher physician fees and a greater degree of service intensity. According to the physician-induced demand and target-income hypotheses, increases in the number of physicians are associated with increases in expenditures for their services. This relationship becomes more important when the interaction of physicians' services and other related health activities is considered. It is estimated that the physician influences approximately 70 percent of total personal health care expenditures.[7] Thus, the number of physicians may be correlated not only with expenditures for physicians' services, but also with expenditures for hospital care, other professional services, and drugs.

Between 1965 and 1981, the number of active physicians increased at an average annual rate of 3.0 percent, nearly triple the 1.1 percent average annual growth rate for the total population. For the period 1981 to 1990, the Bureau of Health Professions projects that the number of active physicians will increase at an average annual rate of 2.7 percent. This increase in the number of physicians is likely to be associated with increases in per capita and aggregate medical expenditures, especially for services that are extensively covered by third-party payments. If insurance pays all costs, a provider's pricing behavior has little effect on consumer demand.[8]

Malpractice Costs

An important cause of higher health expenditures is the increase in malpractice suits filed against physicians. Since attorneys often take these cases on a contingency fee basis, persons with modest incomes are not deterred from filing malpractice cases, while plaintiffs are encouraged to file cases in which they know there is but a small chance of winning. On a national basis, more than 50 percent of all malpractice claims filed are found by the courts to be without merit.

Americans are filing more than three times as many medical claims as they did ten years ago and are obtaining record-breaking settlements. The fear of suits is prompting doctors to order additional tests and treatments, which is adding at least $15 billion annually to total national health expenditures.[9] In each of the last several years, several hundred malpractice awards to patients have exceeded $1 million. After a marked decline in the late 1970s, AMA and insurance industry statistics indicate sixteen malpractice claims were filed for every 100 doctors in 1983, about 20 percent more than the year before, whereas in 1975, fewer than five claims were filed for every 100 doctors. The total value of awards to patients totaled $2 billion in 1983, a 33 percent increase from the figure for 1981.[10]

Malpractice insurance policies can now cost individual physicians up to $80,000 a year, and in several states insurers are presently asking for premium

Table 2–2
Physician Malpractice Claims by
Specialty, 1976–1981

Medical Specialty	Annual Claims per 100 Physicians
All physicians	6.2
Psychiatry	1.9
Pediatrics	3.6
General/family practice	5.1
Anesthesiology	5.2
Internal medicine	5.2
Radiology	5.9
Surgical specialty	9.2
Obstetrics/gynecology	14.0
Other	3.7

Source: U.S. Department of Commerce, *Statistical Abstract, 1985* (Washington, D.C.: U.S. Government Printing Office, 1985), p. 105.

rate increases in excess of 100 percent a year. The impact on services is clear. A survey of 154 Chicago-area physicians who had been sued between 1977 and 1981 found that about one-third of them had stopped performing high-risk procedures, 40 percent had stopped seeing certain kinds of patients, and one-third had considered early retirement.[11]

Table 2–2 shows the considerable difference in the rate of malpractice claims by physician specialty. The rate of claims against specialists in obstetrics/gynecology is more than seven times as high as that against psychiatrists. This may reflect the fact that there is less standardization of therapy in treatment of mental, as opposed to physical, illness. Also, obstetricians are particularly vulnerable because juries are likely to recommend big awards in cases involving infants. Sixty percent of all obstetricians in the United States have been sued, 20 percent of them three or more times. About 25 percent of Florida's obstetricians have stopped practicing their specialty, and another 25 percent plan to stop soon, according to a study by the Florida Obstetric and Gynecologic Society. The primary reason is malpractice liability.[12]

Federal Health Expenditures

From the end of World War II until 1966, public outlays were approximately 25 percent of total expenditures for health and medical care. Expenditures within both the public and private sectors were increasing rapidly but at roughly the same rate. Within the public sector, state and local governments were actually spending more than the federal government. In 1966, the implementation of several major health programs, particularly Medicare and Medicaid, changed these relationships. Public expenditures reached $56.3 billion in 1975 and, thus, represented more than 42 percent of the total. From 1975 to 1982, the proportion of expenditures accounted for by government remained roughly constant although there was a slight decline in 1983. (See table 2–1.) From 1975 to 1983, the federal government accounted for slightly more than two-thirds of all government expenditures for health and medical care; the remainder was from state and local funds. This distribution has fluctuated only slightly in recent years, though in 1965, the year before Medicare and Medicaid were enacted, the federal, state, and local shares were about the same.

Medical Care Inflation

Although the utilization of health services has increased continuously, the major element associated with higher expenditure levels has been rising prices. (See table 2–3.) Thus, from 1965 to 1983, three-fifths of the rise in personal health care expenditures was accounted for by price increases. (Personal health care expenditures account for approximately 90 percent of total national health expenditures.)

Table 2–3
Personal Health Care Expenditures, Average Annual Percentage Change, and Percentage Distribution of Factors Affecting Growth, 1965–1983

Year	Personal Health Care Expenditures (billions of $)	Average Annual Percentage Change	Factors Affecting Growth in Expenditures			
			All Factors	Prices	Population	Intensity
1965–1983		12.7	100	60	9	31
1966	39.6	10.6	100	46	11	43
1968	50.2	13.1	100	43	8	49
1970	65.1	14.5	100	48	8	44
1972	80.2	11.5	100	40	10	50
1974	101.0	13.9	100	66	7	27
1976	131.8	12.9	100	69	8	23
1978	166.7	12.1	100	69	9	22
1980	217.9	15.2	100	75	8	17
1982	286.9	12.7	100	78	8	14
1983	313.3	9.2	100	70	11	19

Source: U.S. Department of Health and Human Services, *Health: United States, 1981*, DHHS Publication No. (PHS) 82-1232 (Washington, D.C.: U.S. Public Health Service, 1982), p. 26.4; Robert Gibson, Daniel Waldo, and Katherine Levit, "National Health Expenditures, 1982," *Health Care Financing Review* 5, no. 1 (Fall 1983):18; Robert Gibson, Katherine Levit, Helen Lazenby, and Daniel Waldo, "Health Care Expenditures, 1983," *Health Care Financing Review* 6, no. 2 (Winter 1984):9.

Historically, medical care prices have increased more rapidly than the price of goods and services in general. For example, during the 1950s, medical care price increases averaged 4 percent annually—nearly twice the rate of increase reported for consumer prices as a whole. During the first half of the 1960s, consumer price increases slowed considerably. The all-items consumer price index (CPI) increased at an average rate of 1.3 percent per annum, while the medical care price index rose 2.5 percent per annum. From 1965 to 1970, prices for goods and services in general rose at an annual rate of 4.2 percent while medical care prices increased 6.1 percent. The implementation of the Medicare and Medicaid programs, which sharply increased the demand for health services without augmenting supply, was partially responsible for the increase in medical prices during that period. From 1970 to 1974, the long standing relationship between CPI (all items) and the medical care price index changed. The average annual rate of increase for the all-items CPI during that time (6.2 percent) was slightly greater than that recorded for the medical care component. This can in part be attributed to the continuous mandatory price controls imposed on the health industry for the duration of the Economic Stabilization Program, which began in August 1971 and ended in April 1974.[13]

From 1974 through 1982 the medical care component of the consumer price index rose an average of 10.2 percent per year, only slightly faster than the 9.1 percent average rise in the CPI. This period of rapid inflation for the economy as a whole reflected the rapid rise in food and energy prices.

Some health economists and others familiar with the health care industry claim that the consumer price index has an upward bias because it fails to take account of quality changes. When the quality of goods deteriorates, the index tends to understate the true price rise; conversely, when quality improves, the index tends to overstate the true rise in the price index. The occurrence of quality changes has always posed problems in calculating price indexes. This is particularly true with prices for medical care and health services, not only because quality changes are especially difficult to measure, but also because quality changes have been rapid. As a result, the view is frequently expressed that the medical care price index may overstate the actual increase in medical care prices. Another limitation of price indexes is the inability of particular items to be representative of an entire grouping of commodities or services. For example, the CPI includes fifteen drugs that have declined slightly in price in recent years. However, newer, more expensive drugs are not included in the index.[14]

As indicated in table 2–3, the importance of inflation as a factor in overall expenditure growth has risen sharply since the mid-1970s, while the significance of intensity (utilization) has declined. The 1974–1981 period was one of rapid inflation generally, and while medical care prices frequently go up more rapidly than consumer prices overall, general inflation does play a major role in terms of total health expenditure increases. Thus, in 1983, 44 percent of the increase in health expenditures was accounted for by general inflation.[15]

It has been suggested that productivity levels in the health services sector are lower than in the overall economy and that the rate of increase in productivity (output per manhour) is slower than in the private sector. Under these conditions, if productivity increases faster in the nonhealth sector than in the health sector, and wages increase at the same rate in both sectors, then unit costs must increase faster in the latter. Statistics on wages, prices, and productivity are consistent with this hypothesis.

Between 1972 and 1981, wages in the health sector increased at an average annual rate of 8.3 percent compared to 7.8 percent in the total private economy. During the period 1969 to 1979, productivity in the health service industry is reported to have actually declined at an average annual rate of 1.4 percent per year, while productivity in the private nonfarm economy increased at an average annual rate of 1.7 percent. For the 1972–1981 period, the medical care services component of the CPI rose at an average annual rate of 9.7 percent compared to the 8.1 percent rate for the overall CPI. Thus, medical care service prices increased at an average annual rate 20 percent faster than overall consumer prices.[16] These calculations used price data rather than unit cost data since the latter were not available for either the health services sector or for the total private economy.

International Comparisons of Health Expenditures

Relatively high rates of growth in health care expenditures are not unique to the United States. Economy-wide inflation, growth in real income, demographic shifts, and rapid technological change have been associated with rising health care costs in the western industrialized countries.

In one study of the rising cost of health care among nine industrialized nations, from 1969 to 1976 expenditures increased at average annual rates ranging from a low of 12.5 percent in the United States, to a high of 20.5 percent in Australia. (See table 2–4.) In all nine countries health expenditures increased as a proportion of GNP. While the United States is among the highest, the Federal Republic of Germany actually was the country with the highest percentage of GNP spent for health care (9.7 percent).

Some analysts suggest that health spending as a proportion of GNP tends to grow in spurts.[17] Countries appear to have relatively effective methods to stem the rise in health spending relative to GNP for a while, but then inefficiency in the system results in sharp health spending increases relative to GNP.

Nations implicitly or explicitly make judgments about the "correct" ratio of GNP allocated to health care. For example, Finland is reported to have

Table 2–4
National Health Expenditures, Selected Industrialized Countries, 1969–1976

Country	Average Annual Rate of Increase 1969–1976 (percent)	As % of GNP 1969	1976
Australia	20.5	5.6	7.7
Finland	18.9	6.0	7.2
Netherlands	18.4	6.0	8.5
United Kingdom	18.2	4.5	5.8
Federal Republic of Germany	17.7	6.3	9.7[a]
France	16.5	6.3	8.2
Sweden	14.6	7.2	8.7[a]
Canada	14.3	6.8	7.1
United States	12.5	7.0	8.7

Source: Mark Freeland and Carol Schendler, "National Health Expenditure Growth in the 1980s: An Aging Population, New Technologies and Increasing Competition," *Health Care Financing Review* 4, no. 3 (March 1983):7.

[a]National health expenditures as percent of gross national product are for 1975.

earmarked 15 percent of GNP for health care under the assumptions that health care is socially desirable and that employment in the health sector is as productive as any other kind of employment.[18]

Health Industry Employment

The health delivery industry is among the largest in the nation. With over 7.2 million employees in 1983, it ranks second in terms of total employment. In 1983 alone, employment in the private health services industry grew three times as fast as that of the private nonfarm economy, whereas health services industry nonsupervisory work hours grew one and one-third times as fast, and nonsupervisory payroll grew one and one-half times as fast. (See table 2–5.) The unemployment rate for health workers was lower than rates for comparably skilled workers in other areas, averaging somewhat more than half the rate of all experienced workers.

The health services industry has been relatively insulated from the business cycle. Since 1972, nonsupervisory work hours in private health establishments have grown an average of 4.9 percent per year. Except for 1983, growth in a single year varied by no more than 1.7 percentage points from the average. In contrast, growth of nonsupervisory work hours in all private nonagricultural establishments averaged 1.2 percent per year, varying in response to the business cycle by as much as 5.7 percentage points in a single year. Growth for the private health industry has been higher and has varied less than growth for the aggregate private nonfarm economy since 1972.[19]

Table 2–5
Measures of Economic Activity in the Health Care Industry and Total U.S. Economy, 1983

Item	Health Care Industry	U.S. Economy
Growth of output or expenditures	10.3	7.7
Growth of constant dollar output or expenditures	3.0	3.7
Growth of total private employment	2.8	0.8
Growth of private nonsupervisory work hours	2.0	1.5
Growth of private nonsupervisory payrolls	8.8	6.0
Civilian unemployment rate	4.6	8.6
Growth of consumer prices	8.7	3.2

Source: Robert Gibson, Katherine Levit, Helen Lazenby, and Daniel Waldo, "National Health Expenditures, 1983," *Health Care Financing Review* 6, no. 2 (Winter 1984):5.

Health Care for Veterans

Aside from Medicare and Medicaid, which are discussed in detail in chapters 4 and 6, the third most costly government-supported health program is that operated by the Veterans Administration.

The Veterans Administration (VA) provides compensation and pensions for military veterans and their survivors, as well as medical care for veterans. Nearly 28.2 million people are eligible to receive some medical care from the VA, although not all of them apply for benefits. In fiscal year 1983, hospital and other medical care for veterans accounted for almost 31 percent of the $24.9 billion in outlays of the VA. In the 1983 National Health Accounts, VA expenditures for personal health care were estimated at $7.6 billion. Of that amount, $6.3 billion, or 83 percent, was spent to provide care in 172 VA medical centers and other hospitals. VA medical centers provided care for 1.3 million inpatients and supplied care during 18.5 million outpatient visits. In fiscal year 1983, 24.3 million inpatient days of care were financed by the Veterans Administration in VA and non-VA hospitals. An additional 9.5 million inpatient days were provided in VA nursing homes or financed by the VA in state- or community-operated nursing facilities.[20]

Between 1980 and 1990, 4.2 million veterans will reach the age of 65. By the year 2000, 63 percent of all American males over 65 will be veterans and, therefore, eligible for VA health services. While the total number of veterans is expected to decline over the next twenty years, the rapid aging of the existing population of veterans has significant cost implications for the VA.[21] It is quite likely that annual increases of $6 billion a year from 1985 to 2000 will be necessary to provide services to the veteran population. In addition, an investment of $6.6 billion over and above current commitments is necessary to provide appropriate health care facilities.[22]

In order to limit future cost increases, the Reagan administration is considering establishing a means test which would deny services to those who could afford private medical care. (See chapter 5.) This measure can be established by regulation and does not require action by Congress. Under such a policy, the government would take into account income from all sources including cash, bank deposits, stock, bonds, and any private health insurance or Medicare coverage available to the veteran. The means test would not apply to veterans who have disabilities connected to their military service, nor would it apply to veterans eligible for Medicaid. Finally, the test would not apply to people receiving veterans' pensions which are paid on the basis of financial need. Under federal law all three groups are assumed to be unable to pay for hospital and nursing home care.[23]

Health Block Grants

During fiscal year 1982, federal block grants were introduced for maternal and child health, preventive health, alcohol/drug rehabilitation, and mental health. A fourth health block grant, primary care, implemented in fiscal 1984, furnishes grants for community health centers to provide care for the medically needy population. Yet total funding has fallen in recent years. A total of $1.1 billion in fiscal year 1981 health expenditures was consolidated into three block grants amounting to only $887 million in fiscal year 1982. This represents an 18 percent decrease in spending. The objective of these block grants is to limit the levels of federal funding and to reduce regulatory involvement while offering states flexibility in responding to their diverse health needs and priorities.[24]

A report to Congress indicates that few program changes occurred during the early part of fiscal year 1982 as a result of the health block grants. States relied on the same mechanisms to handle block grants as were used in the supplanted categorical programs because states had little time or money to institute change. States began to reexamine their needs, prioritize expenditures, and shift funds within the health sector in response to reduced federal funding and to increased state budget constraints.[25]

Programs such as maternal and child health and crippled children's services that affected a broad segment of the population received continued high priority compared with more narrowly defined programs such as the one to prevent lead paint poisoning (which was also included in the maternal and child health block grant). Programs where state involvement was minimal under the old categorical grant system received lower priority under block grants.

Health Status of the American Population

The life expectancy of Americans has improved steadily since 1900, when the average American could expect to live 47.3 years. At that time females lived two more years than males, on an average, and blacks averaged 33.0 years, substantially fewer than the 47.6 year average for whites. By 1982, life expectancy had increased to 74.5 years. The male–female gap had widened to 7.4 years, but the black–white gap had narrowed to less than six years.

The factors primarily responsible for increases in life expectancy during the first half of this century include improved heating and sanitation, better nutrition, and major advances in immunization against infectious diseases. These all greatly contributed to the survival of infants and children. For adults over 65, however, data on additional life expectancy show only modest gains, from 11.9 years in 1900, to 13.9 years in 1950, and 16.8 years in 1982.[26]

Between infancy and age 65 there are distinct differences in major causes of death by age, sex, and race. The leading cause of death for whites and blacks below the age of 15 is accidents. In fact, within the total population, accidents are the leading cause of death below the age of 45. From ages 15 to 24, accidents remain the leading cause of death for whites, whereas homicide is the leading cause of death for blacks. Cancer is the leading cause of death for black females between the ages of 25 and 44, and for white females between the ages of 25 and 64. After age 65, heart disease is the major cause of death.[27]

The major role of accidents and homicides makes clear that behavioral factors play an extremely important role in mortality. Moreover, because many of these deaths occur at early ages, accidents and homicides have a disproportionate effect on life expectancy at birth.

Aside from mortality, another measure of a population's health status is the number of "restricted activity days," which are days that a person reduces his usual activities because of illness or injury. A day spent at home in bed or in the hospital ("bed-disability day") is, of course, a restricted activity day.

Surveys indicate that the number of restricted activity days decreased among all age groups from 1957 until the middle or end of the 1960s, after which the trend shifted. The number of bed-disability days per person fell during the late 1950s and early 1960s and has remained roughly constant since then. Some increase has occurred within the 45 to 64 age group.[28]

Another health status indicator is limitations of activity caused by chronic conditions. A striking trend emerges: the percentage of males aged 45 to 54 who were unable to perform their major activity increased from 7.2 in 1969 to 11.5 percent in 1981. Smaller but very noticeable increases are shown for this activity limitation among other males as well as females aged 45 to 64.

Trends in reported activity limitations may be explained in part by the expansion of disability cash benefits and the number of beneficiaries. Between 1965 and 1975, cash payments to disabled persons increased from $9.7 billion to $33.9 billion. During the same period, the number of social security disability insurance beneficiaries grew by 150 percent, while the covered work force grew by only 55 percent.[29] It appears that persons with chronic conditions can, in recent years, leave the work force with adequate disability benefits, whereas earlier, they might have continued to work. Changes in mortality patterns may also partly explain increases in activity limitations. As mortality rates drop, some people who live longer have chronic diseases that cause disability.

Summary

Although currently growing more slowly than in recent years, total health expenditures continue to account for an increasing share of the gross national product. In 1983, spending for health amounted to 10.8 percent of the gross national product, or $1,459 per person. Public programs financed 40 percent of all personal health spending, a slight decline (in percentage terms) from 1982. Medicare and Medicaid expenditures totaled $91 billion in 1983, or nearly three-tenths of all spending for personal health care.

A major factor in health care expenditure growth is medical price inflation, which has accounted for approximately 70 percent of the increase in health care spending since 1976. One structural cause of medical price inflation is slower growth in productivity within the health care sector as compared to the economy as a whole. Health care expenditures make up approximately the same proportion of GNP in the United States as in most Western European countries in spite of the fact that all Western European countries have national health insurance and the United States does not.

Because of expected rapid gains in Veterans Administration health care costs, the Reagan administration is considering a means test to limit eligibility. Those whose income falls above the limit would no longer be entitled to free care. However, veterans with service-connected disabilities would be exempt from this proposed regulation.

Mortality statistics indicate an enormous improvement in the health status of the American population since 1900 among both sexes, as well as blacks and whites. However, longer life spans have meant that morbidity among some categories of the population has increased, particularly in terms of activity limitations and disability.

Notes

1. Robert Gibson, Katherine Levit, Helen Lazenby, and Daniel Waldo, "National Health Expenditures, 1983," *Health Care Financing Review* 6, no. 2 (Winter 1984):1.

2. M.S. Freeland and Carol Schendler, "Health Spending in the 1980s: Integration of Clinical Practice Patterns with Management," *Health Care Financing Review* 5, no. 3 (Spring 1984):1–68.

3. W.J. Baumol, "Macroeconomics of Unbalanced Growth," *American Economic Review* 57, no. 3 (June 1967):415–26.

4. Robert Gibson and Daniel Waldo, "National Health Expenditures, 1982," *Health Care Financing Review* 5, no. 1 (Fall 1983):17.

5. Congressional Budget Office, *Containing Medical Care Costs through Market Forces* (Washington, D.C.: Congress of the United States, May 1982), p. 26.

6. Bureau of the Census, *Statistical Abstract of the United States, 1982–1983* (Washington, D.C.: U.S. Department of Commerce, 1982), p. 43.

7. Mark Freeland and Carol Ellen Schendler, "National Health Expenditure Growth in the 1980s: An Aging Population, New Technologies and Increasing Competition," *Health Care Financing Review* 4, no. 3 (March 1983):12.

8. Congressional Budget Office, op. cit., p. 28.

9. Sue Miller, "Claims Against Physicians Soar," *The Evening Sun* (Baltimore), January 18, 1985, p. C–1.

10. "Claims Against Doctors Triple," *The Evening Sun* (Baltimore), January 17, 1985, p. A–7.

11. "15 Billion Tag Put on Medical Malpractice Claims," *The Sun* (Baltimore), January 18, 1985, p. 12A.

12. Joanne Lipman, "Huge Malpractice Suits, Premiums Threaten Insurers and Health Care," *Wall Street Journal,* September 21, 1983, section 2, p. 35.

13. U.S. Department of Health, Education, and Welfare, *Medical Care Expenditures, Prices and Costs: Background Book,* DHEW Publication No. (SSA), 75-11909 (Washington, D.C.: U.S. Government Printing Office, 1975), p. 58.

14. Alan Sorkin, *Health Economics: An Introduction,* 2nd ed. rev. (Lexington, Mass.: D.C. Heath, 1984), p. 11.

15. Gibson, Levit, Lazenby, and Waldo, op. cit., p. 9.

16. Freeland and Schendler, op. cit., p. 11.

17. Freeland and Schendler, op. cit., p. 6.

18. "GNP/Health: Can America Determine the Appropriate Relationship?" *Perspective, The Blue Cross and Blue Shield Magazine* (Fall 1982):1–12.

19. Gibson, Levit, Lazenby, and Waldo, op. cit., pp. 4–5.

20. Ibid., p. 24.

21. Veterans Administration, *Caring for the Older Veteran* (Washington, D.C.: U.S. Government Printing Office, 1984), pp. 4–5.

22. Ibid., pp. II–1 to II–6, III–1 to III–3.

23. "New Rules Would Peg Health Benefits for Veterans Under 65 to Income Test," *The Baltimore Sun,* December 20, 1984, pp. 1, 10A.

24. Gibson, Levit, Lazenby, and Waldo, op. cit., pp. 24–25.

25. *Report to Congress: Early Observations on Block Grant Implementation,* GAO/CGO-82-79 (Washington, D.C.: General Accounting Office, 1982).

26. Council of Economic Advisors, *Economic Report of the President, 1985* (Washington, D.C.: U.S. Government Printing Office, 1985), p. 130.

27. Ibid., p. 131.

28. Ibid., p. 131.

29. Ibid., p. 132.

3
Health Manpower

s recently as 1971, the federal government maintained that there was a shortage of at least fifty thousand physicians. While the empirical basis of this shortage estimate was questionable, it served as the single most important reason for the passage of the Comprehensive Health Manpower Training Act of 1971.

This law, which was in effect from 1972 to 1976, was a major piece of health manpower training legislation. It provided four major types of financial assistance to schools and health profession students: construction support, institutional aid, student loans and scholarships, and funding for special programs.

The legislation authorized three kinds of construction assistance: grants, interest subsidies, and loan guarantees. It raised the grant allowable for any project to 70 percent of the total cost, except for expansion programs, in which case grants of 80 percent of cost could be obtained.

The act also provided basic institutional support in the form of capitation payments. To qualify for a capitation grant, each school was required to increase its first year enrollment by a specified percentage. A participating institution received a basic amount for each student, a higher amount for each graduate, and a bonus for students in classes that exceeded the required increased enrollment by 5 percent or five students, whichever was larger.[1]

By 1976, Congressional actions indicated that the overall shortage of physicians had been eliminated. The Health Manpower Act of 1976 removed a number of federal incentives to medical schools to expand physician supply. Moreover, the law considerably restricted the inflow of foreign medical graduates (FMGs) into the United States. The major provisions of the bill were:

1. The federal loan program was replaced by a program of federal loan guarantees. The maximum annual loan a student could receive was $10,000, with a limitation of total indebtedness of $50,000.

2. A small direct-loan program was maintained, but only exceptionally needy students were eligible. Interest rates were increased from 3 to 7 percent.

3. A general program of scholarship support was discontinued. Nearly all scholarships were reserved for persons who joined the National Health Service Corps and thus were serving in federally designated health manpower shortage areas.

4. Each school of medicine, osteopathy, and dentistry received $2,000 in capitation grants in 1978 and $2,100 in 1980. Schools were required to maintain first-year enrollment levels in the following fiscal year and maintain the level of nonfederal expenditures realized the previous year.

5. The 1976 law eliminated immigration preferences for alien graduates of foreign medical schools who had not passed medical qualifying examinations and demonstrated competency in written and oral English. In addition, regulations were developed making it more difficult for foreign medical graduates to obtain exchange visitor visas.[2]

From 1976 to 1984 Presidents Ford, Carter, and Reagan consistently recommended that Congress reduce its funding for health professions education. These recommendations reflected a belief that the supply of many categories of health manpower was adequate if not excessive and, therefore, government subsidies to expand supply were no longer needed. Congress acceded to these cutbacks although at a somewhat slower rate than requested.

Early in 1976 the Secretary of the Department of Health, Education, and Welfare established an advisory committee to review various aspects of graduate medical education. The final report of the Graduate Medical Education National Advisory Committee (GMENAC) was released in September 1980. The GMENAC Report indicated a shortage of physicians in 1978 but projected a growing surplus in a number of specialties.

Year	Demand	Supply
1978	419,000	375,000
1990	466,000	536,000
2000	498,000	643,000

The ratio of physicians to population, which was 171 per 100,000 in 1978, was projected to jump to 220 per 100,000 in 1990, and 247 per 100,000 in 2000.[3]

Moreover, any rapid increase in the number of HMOs would likely add to the potential imbalance between the supply and demand for physicians. This is because HMOs currently employ about 100 physicians per 100,000 persons as compared to an expected national ratio of physicians to population of 250 per 100,000 in 1990. Furthermore, even if one adjusts the HMO figure to compensate for the skewed age distribution of their enrollees (fewer older persons who use more services), a rapid growth of HMOs would significantly reduce the demand for physicians in 1990 and 2000.

Although the projections indicated a substantial overall surplus of physicians by 1990, a number of specialties were still expected to exhibit shortages. (See table 3–1.)

The specialty with the greatest shortage is expected to be psychiatry. Less than 4 percent of today's medical school graduates are undertaking residencies in psychiatry, which limits future supply. Comparatively low incomes of psychiatrists and perhaps some disillusionment with the therapeutic techniques of psychiatry may account for the declining interest among recent medical school graduates in psychiatric residencies.

In order to minimize the expected surplus, the panel recommended three significant actions:

1. Reduce enrollments in American medical schools by 10 to 15 percent. In 1980 there were approximately 70,000 students in the nation's medical schools.

2. Restrict greatly the number of graduates of foreign medical schools who are permitted to practice medicine in the United States. The 40,000 to 50,000 foreign graduates expected to begin practice here in the 1980s account for the bulk of the projected surplus.

3. In view of the aggregate surplus of physicians projected for 1990, medical school graduates in the 1980s should be strongly encouraged to enter those specialties where a shortage of physicians is expected. (See table 3–1.)

Table 3–1
Supply and Requirements, Selected Specialties, 1990

Specialty	Supply	Requirements	Surplus (Shortage)
General psychiatry	30,600	38,500	(7,900)
Emergency medicine	9,250	13,500	(4,250)
Preventive medicine	5,650	7,300	(1,650)
Dermatology	7,350	6,950	400
Family practice	58,200	61,300	(3,100)
Urology	6,050	7,700	(1,650)
Ophthalmology	6,900	11,600	(4,700)
Plastic surgery	3,900	2,700	1,200
General surgery	35,300	23,500	11,800
Neurosurgery	5,100	2,650	2,450
Obstetrics/gynecology	34,450	24,000	10,450
General pediatrics and subspecialties	41,350	36,400	4,950

Source: U.S. Department of Health and Human Services, *Summary Report of the Graduate Medical Education National Advisory Committee*, DHHS Publication No. (HRA) 81-651 (Washington, D.C.: U.S. Government Printing Office, 1980), p. 5.

The panel also recommended that to encourage students to become primary care physicians rather than surgical specialists, the early phase of medical school should emphasize a generalist type of clinical experience and with major emphasis on primary care.

The Omnibus Budget Reconciliation Act of 1981

Partly because of the expected surplus of physicians, and also due to the rising federal budget deficit, the Omnibus Budget Reconciliation Act of 1981 caused federal health manpower expenditures to be cut substantially. Thus, capitation grants to schools of medicine, osteopathy, dentistry, and veterinary medicine were eliminated. Only schools of public health were able to receive such funding for the fiscal years 1982–1984.[4] Financial support for National Health Service Corps scholarships was 40 percent lower in 1982–1984 than in 1980. Moreover, the Omnibus bill sharply reduced the funding for scholarships for the exceptionally needy, with funding 60 percent less in 1982–1984 than in 1980.

This law provided no additional money for construction expenditures on behalf of schools of medicine, osteopathy, dentistry, or veterinary medicine. However, it did permit the Secretary of the Department of Health and Human Services to make all authorized interest subsidy payments on any loan made under these programs prior to October 1, 1981, and provided $4.3 million for fiscal years 1982, 1983, and 1984 to meet these outstanding obligations.[5]

Current Budget Proposals

Continuing this trend of declining support, the 1986 federal budget proposal would eliminate all federal support for training of health profession students who are first-time enrollees. A very small appropriation would be made for students who are in the process of completing training. No funds are made available for construction of health manpower training facilities.

One effect of these budget cuts is that it has become more difficult for young people from low- to moderate-income families to choose a career in one of the health professions. This is especially unfortunate because physicians have tended to come from high-income families even when government assistance to medical students was more generous.

The Impact of a Physician Surplus on the Health Care System

Assuming that the GMENAC projections are reasonably accurate, it is important to consider the probable effects of an expected physician surplus on various aspects of the health care system.

It is not clear how a rapidly increasing supply of physicians will affect health care costs. More physicians could lead to higher overall medical care costs as physicians increase individual utilization rates in order to maintain income in the face of a likely declining patient load. These efforts could result in more surgery, a larger number of follow-up office visits, and more ancillary tests and procedures. To the extent that increases in the physician supply will lead to greater specialization and a wider dispersion of specialists, costs will tend to increase because specialists typically charge more for the same service than do general practitioners. Moreover, an expanded supply of physicians may lead to the substitution of physicians for less costly nonphysician manpower, such as physician assistants.

However, it is conceivable that increased availability of specialists could result in lower overall medical care costs. Specialists, because of their superior training, are less likely to perform questionable medical procedures. They may also tend to make use of fewer tests, feel more secure in treating their patients on an ambulatory basis, and be more expeditious in determining the correct diagnosis and in selecting the most appropriate treatment. This higher level of skill might result in cost savings. Moreover, the expected employment of increasing numbers of physicians in salaried positions by HMOs, group practices, and emergency and urgent care clinics might also contribute to lower costs due to economizing on overhead expenses, reducing individual risk (thereby lowering malpractice insurance rates), and removing incentives to overcharge patients.

New Sources of Demand

Given a much larger supply, physicians are likely to insist on higher standards of medical practice as a means of maintaining or expanding opportunities for employment and earnings. However, it is unclear whether the financial resources required for such quality improvement will be available since the public is unlikely to demand new or improved services if these would result in much larger expenditures.

Still, specific types of patients may be better served. There is, for example, general agreement that many nursing home patients are seriously neglected.[6] Physicians will tend to be more willing to treat elderly patients, especially the very old, whose numbers will increase faster, and whose medical needs are substantially greater than younger patients. Some physicians will be more responsive to meeting the needs of patients who were medically unserved, for example, by establishing practices in low-income neighborhoods and accepting Medicaid patients. This behavior will, to some extent, reflect the increased competition for patients.

A national health insurance program would likely increase the demand for health services and, concomitantly, for various types of medical manpower.

However, given the present federal budget deficit and the rapid increase in the cost of health care, the national health insurance question has become a dead issue.)

Physician-Hospital Relations

Hospital privileges are a vital factor in determining physicians' incomes. This relationship enables physicians to optimize the use of their time, and provides them with a staff-support structure ranging from residents to nurses for their patients. It also enables physicians to charge higher fees for inpatient services.[7] Recent studies by the staff of the American Medical Association tend to confirm the positive influence of hospital privileges on physicians' incomes.

A significant increase in the supply of physicians is likely to have important consequences for physician–hospital relations. It is likely to increase the professional and economic advantages of physicians who hold appointments on the medical staffs of prestigious hospitals. This group of established physicians may tend to limit admitting privileges for younger physicians in order to protect their own volume of work and income. Moreover, as more physicians seek hospital appointments, efforts to reduce bed capacity (in response to declining occupancy rates) may encounter a major source of opposition.

Physician Earnings

A one-third increase in the supply of physicians during a period of highly constrained public and private expenditures for health care is likely to lead to a decline in the average real earnings of physicians. Recent evidence suggests that physicians' incomes have not kept up with those of other professional workers or with the inflation rate. Thus, from 1969 to 1977, physicians' real incomes in the United States fell around 1.75 percent per year.[8] Moreover, from 1982 to 1983, physicians' incomes (unadjusted for inflation) fell 3 percent, primarily due to a 6.2 percent decline in the number of patient visits.[9]

The existence of a larger supply of physicians should make it easier for third-party payers—governmental and nongovernmental alike—to establish systems of fee control whose purpose is to reduce the rate of increase in total health expenditures. The federal government may insist, for example in the case of Medicare, that physicians agree to accept a standard fee and relinquish their current privilege of choosing between direct billing of some Medicare patients while accepting assignments from others.

Lower incomes and fee limitations are likely to change the work patterns of practicing physicians. Some may work more hours per day in order to earn additional income. However, other physicians may decide to adjust their work schedules to the greater convenience of their patients, which would mean more evening or weekend hours. It is not clear which will prove of greater significance, more hours resulting in higher income, or the preference, particularly among younger physicians, for a shorter work week.[10] In all likelihood, the current trend of declining work hours will continue and physicians will work closer to 40 than to 50 hours per week. This trend will be strengthened by the increasing number of physicians who will practice in groups, associations, or in salaried positions as these doctors traditionally work fewer hours per week than solo physicians in private practice.

There has already been a major decline in the number of applicants to dental schools (43 percent since 1975) and osteopathic schools (26 percent since 1976), and a slight decline in applicants to medical schools (15 percent since 1974). The 1984–1985 medical school entering class was down about 1 percent from 1983–1984, the first decline in many years. Given the current reduction in the size of the 18–22 year-old age group and the declining proportion of men attending four-year colleges, a slow or moderate reduction in the number of medical school applicants can be expected. Since many medical school applicants come from the same pool as those who major in engineering and the natural sciences, a movement of many of the better qualified students away from a career in medicine is quite likely if the current strong demand for employment arising from the electronic, energy, and aerospace industries continues. In addition to the prospect of lower lifetime earnings for physicians, the growth of government constraints on practice probably constitutes a major deterrent to some able undergraduates who are considering a medical career.

The Maldistribution of Physicians

Physicians are disproportionately located in the northeast and western regions of the nation as opposed to the southern and north central states. For every 100,000 persons in Mississippi, only 115 physicians provide patient care, a 1:870 ratio. This ratio is contrasted with the 1:333 ratio (300 physicians per 100,000 population) in the state of New York.[11] These ratios reflect a significant deviation from the national average of 206 physicians per 100,000 population, or roughly one physician for every 500 persons. More important, the geographic pattern indicated by these ratios reflects the continued movement of physicians to states and regions with large urban populations. Statistics also indicate that physician/population ratios in states with a relative abundance of physicians are growing slightly faster than such ratios in states with relatively few physicians. (See table 3–2.)

Because the physician supply in nonmetropolitan and metropolitan areas grew at about the same rate during the 1970s, the gap in terms of the physi-

Table 3–2
Active Nonfederal Physicians per 100,000 Population, 1959, 1973, and 1982

	Rate per 100,000 Population		
	1959	1973	1982
Five highest states in 1982			
Five-state average	161	204	289
New York	187	232	300
Massachusetts	174	211	306
Connecticut	162	196	280
Maryland	128	193	300
California	152	190	258
Five lowest states in 1982[a]			
Five-state average	77	86	131
South Dakota	68	75	131
Mississippi	72	82	120
Arkansas	88	89	140
Alabama	74	91	139
Idaho	83	92	124

Source: Department of Health, Education, and Welfare, *Health Manpower Source Book*, section 10, "Physician's Age, Type of Practice, and Location," PHS Publication No. 263 (Washington, D.C.: U.S. Government Printing Office, 1960) p. 14; American Medical Association, *Physician Characteristics and Distribution in the United States*, 1974, pp. 26 and 39, and 1983, pp. 31 and 45.

[a]Alaska has only 134 nonfederal physicians per 100,000 persons, but was excluded from the table because of the large number of physicians employed by the Public Health Service.

cian/population ratio (about 2.3:1) between these areas remained unchanged during the decade. However, the 35 percent growth in nonmetropolitan areas represented a significant improvement in physician supply over past levels. Physician supply had grown only 11 percent during the 1960s, which was less than one-third the growth rate in metropolitan counties. The increase during the 1970s was greatest in the more isolated rural areas. While physician supply in rural areas actually declined 11 percent during the 1960s, between 1974 and 1978 it rose 23 percent, which was actually more than the national rate.[12]

Yet, at the end of 1982, there were 131 counties in the United States that had no active physicians in patient care. This compared to 139 such counties in 1977. These 131 counties cover 118,568 square miles or approximately 3.4 percent of the total U.S. land area. Slightly more than one-half million (500,400) people (0.21 percent of the total U.S. population) reside in these counties. The most populous county (23,800) was Meade, Kentucky, while Esmeralda County, Nevada, with 1,500 inhabitants occupies the largest area, 3,587 square miles.[13]

The effect of this physician shortage is clear. There is more chronic disease and there are more days of work lost per person in nonmetropolitan than in metropolitan counties. Among nonmetropolitan residents, 47.4 percent have one or more chronic conditions, compared with 44.9 percent for urban residents.[14] The disparity is larger for activity-limiting chronic conditions: about 15 percent of nonmetropolitan residents suffer from them, compared with 10.5 percent for metropolitan residents.[15] Although infant mortality rates are about the same on the average in nonmetropolitan and metropolitan counties, all counties with an infant mortality rate at least double the national rate are nonmetropolitan, and 80 percent of these are in the most rural group. Thus, the localities with the greatest need for physicians have the greatest shortages.

A recent study of physician location trends indicated that between 1960 and 1977 there was a substantial movement of board-certified specialists from the large metropolitan centers into smaller communities, probably in response to increased competition for patients in urban areas. Thus, more than 70 percent of all towns of 20,000 to 30,000 population now have a full complement of basic specialists.[16] The rising number of new graduates will likely reinforce these trends until the point is reached where most small communities will have as many primary care physicians and specialists as can earn an adequate income. It is of interest that this large-scale movement of physicians into smaller towns and cities occurred at precisely the same time that the issue of physician maldistribution was of such intense concern to both medical and political leaders.

Two additional events reflect the large-scale movement of specialists into outlying areas. First, major university hospitals have been experiencing a reduced flow of patients coming from small- and medium-sized communities to obtain secondary and frequently even tertiary care. These localities used to provide many referrals to these metropolitan hospitals because the former lacked the specialists to treat patients in their home communities. Moreover, university hospitals located in metropolitan areas have been admitting progressively fewer suburban patients. In both cases, the diffusion of specialists is the major cause of the declining transfer of patients into major medical centers.

Moreover, for-profit hospital chains have been active recruiters of key specialists such as orthopedic surgeons, anesthesiologists, and radiologists. These personnel are necessary to ensure that the medical staffs in their outlying hospitals have sufficient breadth and depth to maintain high utilization rates.

Given the changing location of specialists, one should consider the implications and consequences of an increasing number of them establishing practices in smaller communities. How will family practitioners who are presently disproportionately concentrated in such locations be affected economically as a result of such a continuing movement? Underutilized general practitioners may be more reluctant to refer their patients to specialists, particularly if these GPs are suffering declines in income.

There is one element of caution that must be considered in all discussions concerning the degree of maldistribution of health care. The analyst must not limit consideration to only one dimension of health manpower or services. He should consider the full range of health personnel in a locale before reaching conclusions about the maldistribution of health care workers. The ratio of physicians to population may be relatively low in a particular area, but when nurses and other health personnel are considered, the same area may be considered relatively well-supplied. Moreover, one must remember that reducing the maldistribution of health manpower would not by itself assure an equality in the provision of health services. A community requires not only health manpower, but also facilities, equipment, and most importantly, a health delivery mechanism if all the members of the community are to receive a reasonable amount and quality of health care. Manpower alone does not directly translate into services.

Foreign Medical Graduates

The 1976 Health Manpower Act has reduced the rate of FMG inflow somewhat less than its supporters had expected. The most recent data indicate 96,605 FMGs are in medical practice in the United States, accounting for 21 percent of all physicians.[17] While there was a decline in the number of FMGs in house officer positions in the late 1970s, their proportion of all house staff seems to have stabilized at 19 percent by 1982–1983. (See table 3–3.)

Moreover, there is the continuing situation of U.S. FMGs who obtain degrees from overseas medical schools and return to the United States to enter

Table 3–3
House Officers in the United States, 1961–1962 to 1982–1983

Training Year	All House Officers	FMG House Officers	FMGs as a % of All House Officers
1961–1962	37,810	8,996	23.8
1965–1966	41,568	11,474	27.6
1970–1971	51,015	16,282	31.9
1974–1975	62,512	18,115	29.0
1976–1977	60,651	15,097	24.9
1978–1979	63,163	12,821	20.3
1979–1980	64,615	12,070	18.7
1980–1981	61,465	12,078	19.7
1981–1982	68,217	13,194	19.3
1982–1983	69,142	13,123	19.0

Source: Adapted from Stephen Mick and Jacqueline Worobey, "Foreign Medical Graduates in the 1980s: Trends in Specialization," *American Journal of Public Health* 74, no. 7 (July 1984):699.

house officer programs. Until very recently, in order to qualify for a house officer position, U.S. FMGs needed only to pass the older ECFMG examination instead of the more difficult Visa Qualifying Examination given to FMGs who were non-U.S. citizens. The easier examination may have contributed to an increasing inflow of U.S. FMGs into the country. (See table 3–4.)

In the early 1970s, the fraction of FMG house officers that were U.S. FMGs was 5–8 percent. This figure rose to 48.7 percent in 1982–1983. Subtracting the U.S. FMGs from the combined FMG pool leaves, in each of the four years beginning 1979–1980, 7,841, 7,288, 7,356, and 6,735 alien FMGs respectively. Thus, while the number of U.S. FMGs increased over this period from 4,229 to 6,388, the decline in the number of alien FMGs appears to have moderated.[18]

Given that FMGs continue to significantly add to the total supply of U.S. physicians, the likelihood of a substantial surplus by 1990 as projected by the GMENAC report seems increasingly likely. However, changes in FMG testing may affect the number of FMGs obtaining house officer positions in the United States. The new Foreign Medical Graduate Examination in the Medical Sciences replaced the two examinations given to alien FMGs and U.S. FMGs in July 1984, and was designed to evaluate the knowledge of all FMGs in the basic and clinical sciences. Whether this new two-day examination will further reduce the number of alien FMGs and discourage overseas medical studies by U.S. citizens is yet to be determined.

Table 3–4
Number of U.S. FMGs and U.S. FMGs as a Percent of All FMGs by Year, 1971–1972 to 1982–1983

Year	Number of U.S. FMGs	U.S. FMGs as a % of All FMGs
1971–1972	699	5.3
1972–1973	657	3.6
1973–1974	1,198	6.5
1974–1975	1,738	9.6
1975–1976	1,466	8.7
1976–1977	2,820	18.7
1977–1978	3,361	24.5
1978–1979	3,902	30.4
1979–1980	4,229	35.0
1980–1981	4,790	39.7
1981–1982	5,838	44.2
1982–1983	6,388	48.7

Source: Adapted from Stephen Mick and Jacqueline Worobey, "Foreign Medical Graduates in the 1980s: Trends in Specialization," *American Journal of Public Health*, 74, no. 7 (July 1984):700.

Recent Developments in Licensing Foreign Medical Graduates

Partly in response to the expected surplus of physicians, states are becoming increasingly restrictive in terms of awarding licenses to FMGs, particularly those who are U.S. citizens who obtained medical degrees from diploma mills.

Maryland's medical examiners recently refused to license fourteen newly graduated doctors with degrees from two medical schools, one in the Caribbean and one in Mexico. The Maryland examiners explained the refusal by saying their concern is the welfare of the patients.

In 1983–1984, California rejected 30 percent of all FMGs seeking licenses because of "major deficiencies" in training or documentation.[20] Unfortunately there is evidence that these persons are practicing medicine in states with less stringent licensing requirements or have joined what is sometimes called a "medical underground."

Dr. Ray Casterline of the Educational Council for Foreign Medical Graduates estimates that several hundred graduates of "diploma-mill" medical schools have found their way into American medicine. Four schools in the Dominican Republic gave 2,100 false degrees to would-be doctors who paid intermediaries up to $50,000 each. Many of these buyers never saw the schools, or even the Caribbean, until graduation.

Even standardized testing of these people has not proven to be an adequate safeguard. In July 1983, 17,600 persons took the Educational Council's test for foreign graduates who seek U.S. hospital internships or residencies as a prelude to licensing. Officials soon discovered that 3,000 to 4,000 applicants, the majority Americans, had bought or seen the answers. The test had been stolen and sold for amounts ranging from $5,000 to $50,000.[21]

The problem of diploma-mill medical schools appears most acute in the Dominican Republic. This small nation has fourteen medical schools, an increase of ten in the past ten years. Many of these schools are little more than a few classrooms. They often have no hospital affiliation and minimal laboratory and library facilities. Many give their students two years or less in the classroom, and then send them to two-year "clerkships" in American hospitals, often small ones without university affiliation that are unable to attract students from U.S. medical schools to the housestaff.

Clearly strong measures are needed to guarantee the quality of foreign medical school graduates seeking to practice in the U.S. It is difficult to exaggerate the importance of this issue.

Nurses

There has been a great increase in the number of active registered nurses in recent decades—from 335,000 in 1950 to 1,452,000 in 1982, including both full- and part-time nurses. Computing the full-time equivalency of the part-time nurse work-force indicates a full-time equivalent of 1,234,000 active registered nurses in 1982, or 534 full-time equivalent nurses per 100,000 population.[22] This increase has been stimulated by continuous federal support of nursing schools for nearly thirty years.

Projections indicate a continued rise in the number of nurses to 1990 although the rate of increase will be below that of recent decades. There will be 1,509,000 active nurses in 1990, a ratio of 617 per 100,000 population. The number of full-time equivalent nurses projected for 1990 is 1,272,000, representing a ratio of 540 per 100,000.[23]

In the early 1980s, it was common among physicians, nurses, and some political leaders to claim that there was a shortage of registered nurses (RNs). However, economists generally disagreed and argued that the apparent shortage in hospitals, where 60 percent of nurses are employed, was caused by the facts that RNs' salaries were too low and that the monopsonistic nature of the nurse labor market as regards hospital employment causes an exaggeration of the nurse vacancy rate. Their salaries were rising more slowly than those of lesser trained licensed practical nurses, while at the same time, the income gap between registered nurses and physicians was growing.

The tremendous growth in the supply of nurses has acted to hold down their wages. As their supply has increased, demand has not been maintained despite the growing complexity of medicine and the increased intensity of nursing care per day of hospital care. This is because the length of the hospital stay has fallen and in recent years the occupancy rate has declined.[24]

As an example of this shift, the number of unfilled nursing jobs in Maryland hospitals dropped from 13.8 percent in 1980, to 6.1 percent in 1984. In the Baltimore area, it dropped from 14.8 percent to 6 percent.[25] The reduced vacancy rate is not the result of a large increase in supply since supply is merely growing slowly. The decline in vacancies is due to a drop in demand for hospital nurses, reflecting the impact of the recessions of 1980 and 1981–1982 on hospital visits, as well as the increased competition facing hospitals from other health care providers.

Unfavorable hours, night and weekend shifts, pay that is lower than that for jobs with similar requirements, increased stress (especially in intensive care units), and dissatisfaction with status make hospital nursing a relatively unattractive profession for college-educated women and men. Given the increased job opportunities for college-educated women in higher paying fields, the academic ability of those who will enter nursing will likely fall, while the wages of nurses will lag behind those of people in other fields with comparable levels of formal education.

The fact that government and other third parties are currently increasing their efforts at cost containment increases the likelihood of a reduced flow of additional resources into the health care industry, particularly into hospitals.

This implies a weakening demand for nurses. However, two factors could result in increased demand for nurses: advancing knowledge and technology, and the rise of nurse practitioners to provide primary care to particular groups of underserved patients. Yet, before examining these potentialities more closely, it is essential to consider cost-containment strategies.

Concerning long-term care, certain factors are of importance. Nursing homes have expanded rapidly during the past decade, and they are staffed primarily by nursing personnel below the level of the registered nurse. There are no comprehensive studies of the quality of care provided in various long-term care institutions, but health care experts believe that much of it is at less than an acceptable level. The increased employment of registered nurses, in addition to or as substitutes for personnel now employed, could probably contribute to an improved level of care. However, this upgrading in personnel would be difficult to finance. Medicaid payments are being reduced, and the consumer is presently paying approximately one-half the total costs of nursing home care.

Despite occasional successes in a few states, nurses have recently experienced considerable resistance as they have attempted to broaden the scope of nurse practice acts.[26] The GMENAC report recommended that, with minor exceptions, physician extenders (nurse practitioners and physicians assistants) must continue work under the supervision of doctors, and that their supply not be increased. However, groups of health auxiliaries will attempt to increase their scope of responsibility and their degree of independence from physician supervision. Moreover, there will be a continuing need among such special groups as the isolated and the poor for coverage by physician extenders where physician services will not be available.

The recent revision of federal immigration regulations to greatly reduce the inflow of foreign nurse graduates reflects a broad agreement among government officials, nursing organizations, and employers that the number of domestically trained nurses is adequate to meet the present and future market demand. If the new regulations succeed in substantially reducing the immigration of foreign graduates (currently about 8,000 per annum), it may reduce the probability of a surplus among American nurses.[27]

Physician Assistants and Nurse Practitioners

Physician organizations are likely to become increasingly restrictive regarding the number of physician extenders being trained as well as their approved scope of practice. This will be especially the case if the expected surplus of physicians actually occurs.

In all states where the licensure boards consist primarily of physicians, the *independent* practice of medicine by physician assistants is illegal. All states prohibit the practice of "medicine" by anyone who is not a physician. However, the line between what constitutes nursing practice and medical practice has become blurred and some physician extenders are able to work under the nursing practice acts. Since 1971, thirty-eight states have amended laws to allow nurses to diagnose, prescribe drugs, and perform other duties that were once prohibited to them by the Medical Practice Acts.[28] These functions are beyond traditional nursing activities and therefore directly affect the demand for physicians' services.

The expansion of physician extenders' roles will have a major impact on health care costs. Traditionally, strict licensure rules and union practices have limited the number of persons who could perform a given function, thus driving up hospital and other institutional costs. Smaller hospitals cannot fully utilize their technical personnel when each individual is licensed to perform only a specific task, which reduces hospital productivity and efficiency. If the quality of medical services is not harmed by the removal of such restrictive work rules, then their elimination is in the public interest.

In February 1978, the federal government acted to increase competition on the supply side of the health care market by directly reimbursing personnel such as general nurse practitioners who treat Medicare patients.[29] However, federal legislation does not override the state professional practice acts, and direct reimbursement of physician extenders is limited to those working in rural and selected urban areas. If general nurse practitioners were reimbursed directly by all insurers, their use would be greatly increased. These health care workers seem especially suitable to make home care visits to the chronically ill. Legislation in 1980 eliminated the prior hospitalization requirement for Medicare reimbursement of home health care. Home visits are believed to be a cost-effective activity because they postpone, and for some individuals eliminate, the need for nursing homes, a more expensive and generally less desirable option.

In 1985, there were about 40,000 physician assistants and general nurse practitioners, a number that is likely to grow because of the existence of about 250 educational programs for various types of physician extenders. About 15,000 nurses of all kinds are in independent practice. Approximately 2,000 of these are midwives, some are public health nurses serving the chronically ill in their homes, and others treat the poor in health clinics. Although the new independence of the more highly educated nurses is being challenged, primarily by physicians, the upgrading of nurses for expanded roles is likely to continue throughout the 1980s.[30]

Estimates of the increase in productivity of physicians derived from hiring additional aides range from 50 percent to 75 percent. Because the salaries of physician assistants and nurse practitioners are only about one-third of physicians' earnings, their cost-effectiveness after allowances for capital costs of office space and equipment and costs of supervision is substantial. However, costs to the consumer are reduced only if the savings are passed on to the consumer, and not added to the profits of the physician or the groups that hire physicians and physician extenders.

Summary

As the various branches of the federal government have perceived an end to the physician shortage, support for medical education has been reduced. Indeed, in the president's 1986 budget such funding has been virtually eliminated. Moreover, the GMENAC report forecasts a substantial surplus of physicians by 1990 and, in the absence of offsetting policies, an even larger surplus by the year 2000. However, some specialties such as general psychiatry and emergency medicine will remain in short supply.

This physician surplus has a number of implications. These include possible reductions in the relative earnings of physicians and in the length of their work week; a continuing decline in the maldistribution of physicians as more of them practice in small towns and rural areas; increased restriction of hospital privileges; and a greater willingness of physicians to treat the poor and thus accept Medicaid patients.

The Health Manpower Act of 1976 contained provisions to reduce the flow of foreign medical graduates into the U.S. health care system. These restrictions have been only partially successful, thus increasing the likelihood that a surplus of physicians will actually occur. Nearly one-half of all FMGs presently obtaining house staff positions are U.S. citizens who went overseas to study medicine.

Several states are becoming less willing to license foreign medical graduates, particularly those who are U.S. citizens. There is evidence that some medical schools in Mexico and the Caribbean are diploma mills providing grossly inadequate training or no training at all.

The rapid increase in the supply of nurses has eliminated the general nurse shortage. Moreover, the pressure from both federal and state governments, as well as third-party payers for cost containment, combined with declining hospital occupancy rates is reducing the demand for registered nurses.

The number of physician extenders (particularly nurse practitioners and physician assistants) has grown rapidly for the past twenty years. Because of expansion in the nursing practice acts, nurses are able to perform functions that once were restricted to physicians. However, it is likely that physician organizations will attempt to limit the number of physician extenders being trained, as well as the kinds of tasks they are permitted to perform.

Notes

1. Louise Russell, Blair Bourque, and Carol Burke, *Federal Spending, 1969–1974* (Washington, D.C.: National Planning Association, 1974), p. 28.

2. U.S. Congress, *Congressional Quarterly Almanac, 1976* (Washington, D.C.: U.S. Government Printing Office, 1976), pp. 2685–87.

3. Graduate Medical Education National Advisory Committee, *GMENAC Summary Report to the Secretary, Department of Health and Human Services*, vol. 1 (Washington, D.C.: U.S. Department of Health and Human Services, 1980), p. 3.

4. Association of American Medical Colleges, *The Omnibus Budget Reconciliation Act of 1981*, Memorandum 81-37, August 7, 1981, processed, attachment II, p. 1.

5. Association of American Medical Colleges, *op. cit.*, attachment II, p. 10.

6. Bruce Vladeck, *Unloving Care: The Nursing Home Tragedy* (New York: Basic Books, 1980), pp. 7–29.

7. Mark Pauly, *Doctors and Their Workshops* (Chicago: National Bureau of Economic Research, 1980), pp. 17–24.

8. Jacques Van Der Gaag and Mark Perlman, eds., *Health, Economics, and Health Economics, Proceedings of the World Congress on Health Economics, Leiden, Netherlands, September 1980* (New York: North Holland, 1981), p. 94.

9. Cristine Russell, "Getting the Patients In," *The Washington Post*, November 12, 1984, p. A-3.

10. Eli Ginzberg, Edward Brann, Dale Hiestand, and Miraim Ostow, "The Expanded Physician Supply and Health Policy: The Clouded Outlook," *Milbank Memorial Fund Quarterly/Health and Society*, 59, no. 4 (Fall 1981):521.

11. *Physician Characteristics and Distribution in the United States, 1982* (Chicago: American Medical Association, 1983), p. 34.

12. *Third Report to the President and Congress on the Status of Health Professions in the United States*, DHHS Publication No. (HRA) 82-2 (Washington, D.C.: U.S. Department of Health and Human Services, 1982), p. iv–96.

13. *Physician Characteristics*, p. 68.

14. U.S. Department of Health, Education, and Welfare, *Health Characteristics by Geographic Region, Large Metropolitan Areas and Other Places of Residence—U.S., July 1963–June 1965*, series no. 10, no. 36, National Center for Health Statistics (Washington, D.C.: U.S. Government Printing Office, 1967), pp. 18, 22, 28, 34.

15. U.S. Department of Agriculture, Economics Research Service, *Rurality, Poverty and Health: Medical Problems in Rural Areas*, Agricultural Economic Report no. 172 (Washington, D.C.: U.S. Government Printing Office, 1970), pp. 21–22.

16. W.B. Schwartz, J.P. Newhouse, B.W. Bennett, and A.P. Williams, "The Changing Distribution of Board Certified Physicians," *New England Journal of Medicine* 303 (1980):1032–38.

17. Stephen Mick and Jacqueline Worobey, "Foreign Medical Graduates in the 1980s: Trends in Specialization," *American Journal of Public Health*, 74, no. 7 (July 1974):698.

18. Mick and Worobey, op. cit., p. 700.

19. Educational Commission for Foreign Medical Graduates and National Board of Medical Examiners. *Announcement: FMG Examination in the Medical Sciences,* January 17, 1983 (Washington, D.C.: Educational Commission for Foreign Medical Graduates).

20. Victor Cohn, "Qualifications of New Doctors Challenged," *The Washington Post,* June 3, 1984, p. A-3.

21. Ibid.

22. U.S. Department of Commerce, *Statistical Abstract of the United States, 1983–1984* (Washington, D.C.: U.S. Government Printing Office, 1984), p. 109.

23. *Supply of Manpower in Selected Health Occupations, 1950–1990,* DHHS Publication No. (HRA) 80-35 (Washington, D.C.: U.S. Department of Health and Human Services, 1980), pp. 58, 62.

24. Rita Ricardo-Campbell, *The Economics and Politics of Health* (Chapel Hill: The University of North Carolina Press, 1982), p. 61.

25. Susan Warner, "Once in Demand, Nurses Now Facing Prospect of Fewer Jobs," *The Evening Sun* (Baltimore), December 28, 1984, p. A-1.

26. T.M. Trandel-Korunchuck and K. Trandel-Korunchuck, "Current Legal Issues Facing Nursing Practice," *Nursing Administration Quarterly* 5 (1980):1.

27. Eli Ginzberg, "Policy Directions," in Michael Mellman, ed., *Nursing Personnel and the Changing Health Care System* (Cambridge, Mass.: Ballinger Publishing Co., 1978), p. 265.

28. "For 'New Nurse': Bigger Role in Health Care," *U.S. News and World Report,* January 14, 1980, p. 60.

29. Ricardo-Campbell, op. cit., p. 54.

30. Ibid., p. 55.

4
Medicare

T he Medicare program is designed to finance acute medical care mainly
for elderly Americans. The program is divided into two parts: Part
A, which is hospital insurance (HI), and Part B, which is supplementary medical insurance (SMI). The HI component covers short-term hospitalization, skilled nursing care, and home health services; while the SMI portion
covers physicians' services, outpatient hospital care, and laboratory fees, as
well as home health care. The program does not cover long-term nursing
home care, dental care, or outpatient drugs.

Cost sharing is imposed on Medicare beneficiaries who use medical services. Under HI, a deductible amount approximately equal to the cost of one
day in a hospital ($400 in 1985) must be paid by beneficiaries who are
hospitalized. Aside from this deductible, the HI program pays in full the cost
of the first sixty days of hospitalization for an episode of illness. From the
sixty-first day through the ninetieth days, a 25 percent coinsurance payment
of $100 per day is required as of 1985. For stays of more than ninety days,
each beneficiary has a life-time reserve of sixty additional days but must pay
$200 for each day that is used.[1]

HI also covers up to one hundred posthospital days in a skilled nursing
facility (SNF). After twenty days, the beneficiary is required to pay an
amount per day that is equal to 12.5 percent of the inpatient hospital deductible ($50 in 1985).

Under SMI, as of 1985 beneficiaries must pay $15.50 per month plus an
annual deductible of $75, beyond which Medicare pays 80 percent of the
"reasonable charges" for covered services. If the provider's charges are reasonable according to Medicare standards, then the patient's share is the remaining 20 percent of the total. If the charges exceed such standards, the
beneficiary is liable for the excess amount in addition to his 20 percent share
(except when the physician accepts assignment).

State Medicaid programs frequently serve to complement Medicare for
low-income elderly persons. Medicaid may finance cost-sharing amounts as

well as other noncovered services for eligible Medicare beneficiaries who are too poor to pay these bills.

There are several justifications for Medicare's cost-sharing provisions. First, cost sharing reduces the cost of the program to the federal government. Since the program must be financed through taxes or other revenues, the absence of cost-sharing provisions would lead to higher taxes or less money available for other federal programs. The use of deductibles and coinsurance thus permits Medicare to cover more services than otherwise.

Second, cost sharing makes the consumer aware of the cost of services, thus limiting unnecessary utilization. Deductibles and coinsurance provide both patients and physicians with an incentive to choose the most cost-effective forms of care. Without cost sharing, activities to constrain volume would be almost exclusively carried out by regulatory agencies.

Finally, the high deductible feature of the HI program encourages patients to obtain outpatient treatment instead of inpatient hospital care. This assumes, of course, that the patient has an illness which can be appropriately treated on an outpatient basis and that he has the motivation to obtain that type of care. It also assumes that such care is available. The deductible is also intended to deter unnecessary use of skilled nursing facilities. Since elderly people are most likely to suffer from chronic conditions, there is a tendency to admit them into SNFs even though custodial care is more appropriate. A three-day hospitalization is required before a beneficiary becomes eligible for SNF benefits. This is done to discourage the use of SNFs for custodial purposes.

While cost sharing may reduce utilization, it may also discourage patients from getting medically necessary services. Thus, constraints on utilization could negatively impact on an individual's health status and lower the quality of care received. Because of cost sharing, patients may postpone treatment until an illness becomes so severe that the total cost of care is much greater than would have been the case if they had received prompt treatment. Similarly, physicians may do less diagnostic testing on patients with high deductibles or coinsurance. Yet, early diagnosis may result in effective treatment at relatively low cost.

A second major criticism of cost sharing relates to the issue of equity. A uniform deductible or coinsurance places a greater relative burden on the poor than on high-income families. However, if cost sharing is related to family income levels, it becomes complex and expensive to administer the program.

Finally, cost sharing will cause some individuals to purchase supplementary insurance in order to reduce their out-of-pocket medical expenses. This will likely reduce any effects on the demand for services that cost sharing is expected to achieve.

The empirical evidence strongly suggests that coinsurance significantly reduces utilization of health services. Most studies conclude that the greater the out-of-pocket cost to consumers, the fewer services—particularly out-patient physicians' services—they will demand. For example, Scitovsky and Snyder examined the utilization patterns of subscribers to a medical plan before and after a 25 percent coinsurance provision was instituted. They determined that utilization of physician services per subscriber fell by 24 percent after the coinsurance provisions took effect.[2] In a follow-up study Scitovsky and McCall found that the lower use rates, which occurred soon after the coinsurance took effect, were maintained during subsequent years, indicating that the initial impact was not a short-term phenomenon.[3]

A recent, generalized study concerning the effect of coinsurance on utilization is reported by Newhouse et al.[4] It was found that per capita expenditures for inpatient and ambulatory services rose steadily as the coinsurance rate declined. Persons receiving free care incurred expenditures that were about 60 percent higher than did people whose coverage was limited to catastrophic expenditures. Newhouse found no evidence to support Roemer's conclusion that high-deductible plans are ultimately more expensive because they result in neglect of illnesses and thus are associated with higher hospitalization rates. In fact, the former found the probability of hospitalization was highest for persons who did not pay for care. Finally, it was concluded that the poor were not disporportionately affected by cost sharing, although they would have been had the cost sharing not been related to family income.

While these studies do not consider effects of coinsurance or deductibles on the utilization of health services by the elderly, the Medicare program itself does provide evidence concerning the effect of price changes on utilization. Before Medicare was enacted, only about one-third of the elderly had health insurance coverage. Those who were uninsured faced financial problems when they became seriously ill, and many elderly persons were forced to rely on charity care. In all probability some uninsured elderly individuals delayed seeking necessary medical treatment. When Medicare became law, the average utilization rate among the elderly increased immediately by over 30 percent. The average number of physician visits per elderly person rose by more than 40 percent. These higher utilization rates have been maintained up to the present.[5]

A major weakness of Medicare's benefit structure is that it violates the primary purpose of insurance, which is to protect the beneficiary from destitution. The cost-sharing provisions of the HI and SMI mean that elderly people face unlimited liabilities if a catastrophic illness occurs. Under HI, patients are required to pay the entire hospital cost after 150 days of hospitalization. Moreover, they have already paid relatively high coinsurance rates beginning on the ninety-first day. Furthermore, SMI requires patients to pay 20 percent of reasonable charges for physician visits as well as other outpatient services. For expensive surgery, the 20 percent coinsurance rate could be a costly financial burden on an elderly patient. Consequently, even though the probability of a large financial outlay is low, there is an incentive for beneficiaries to buy supplementary insurance coverage. This weakness in Medicare's benefit structure helped to create the demand for what is presently called Medigap insurance.[6]

Medigap insurance pays a substantial portion of the health care costs that are not covered by Medicare. It permits those elderly persons who can afford this insurance roughly the same degree of insurance protection as that obtained by employed nonaged persons.

A second major difficulty associated with Medicare cost-sharing provisions is that they were designed under the assumption that beneficiaries will have adequate information about the relative cost of services offered by different providers as well as the variety of health care facilities available. In fact, patients have limited knowledge regarding the fees charged by physicians and the prices charged by hospitals and clinics. Such information is not easy to obtain. More important, since it is usually the physician who makes the decision about what tests should be done, what procedures should be performed, and where the patient should be hospitalized, the patient's influence concerning the course of treatment is limited.

Medicare Cost Controls

As table 4–1 indicates, both overall national health costs and Medicare costs have been rising rapidly since enactment of the latter in 1965. In 1983, Medicare's HI costs were almost eight times the 1970 level, and SMI costs were more than six times the amount spent in 1970. Over the same period, non-Medicare hospital costs (total costs less expenditures under Medicare's HI) rose nearly seven times, and costs of non-Medicare physicians' services almost quintupled. Some of the difference in the rates of increase in total costs is due to the growth and aging of the elderly population. The difference also results from covering the disabled and persons with end-state renal disease under Medicare after 1972. Increases in Medicare utilization rates and prices explain only a small portion of the differential expenditure growth.

Cost Containment Legislation

In order to increase controls on utilization, the Professional Standards Review Organization (PSRO) program was enacted in 1972. Provisions were also adopted to limit increases in physicians' fees allowed by Medicare, with increases to be controlled by an index. Furthermore, the legislation authorized cost limits to be applied in determining which costs incurred by hospitals could be reimbursed.

Table 4–1
National Health Expenditures, Hospital and Physician Insurance Expenditures, and Medicare Expenditures, 1960–1983[a]
(billions of dollars)

	Total Health Expenditures	Percentage of GNP	Hospital Insurance	Insurance for Physicians Services	Total Medicare	Medicare Hospital Insurance	Supplementary Medical Insurance
1960	$ 26.9	5.3	$ 5.7	$ 2.0	—	—	—
1965	41.7	6.0	13.9	8.5	—	—	—
1970	74.7	7.5	27.8	14.3	$ 7.4	$ 5.3	$ 2.1
1975	132.7	8.6	52.1	24.9	16.0	11.6	4.4
1980	249.0	9.5	100.4	46.8	36.8	25.6	10.7
1981	286.6	9.8	118.0	54.8	43.6	30.7	12.9
1982	322.3	10.3	134.9	61.8	51.1	36.7	11.4
1983	355.4	10.8	147.2	69.0	57.8	40.4	13.4

Source: Robert Gibson, Katherine Levit, Helen Lazenby, and Daniel Waldo, "National Health Expenditures, 1983," *Health Care Financing Review* 6, no. 2 (Winter 1984):1,7–8, 17, 20–21.
[a]For periods ending June 30.

Despite the legislative controls on physician fee increases, SMI costs have continued to rise rapidly because of volume increases and the ineffectiveness of the controls. The physician fee limitation was applied without developing a federal definition of the various services subject to fee limitation. As a result, some bypassing of controls occurred due to the introduction of new services, and changes in the content of services, including so-called "unbundling" (submitting separate charges for parts of a service that were previously billed as a unit).

One of the problems associated with greater controls on physician fees is that if the physician bills the patient rather than billing Medicare, the physician can charge any amount he deems appropriate, in effect shifting more of the costs of Medicare-covered services to the patient. This change in billing practice has tended to slowly reduce the portion of the beneficiary costs covered by Medicare, thus preventing the imposition of more stringent controls on physician fees by program administrators.

At the same time that physician fee payments were constrained by the index, a limit was placed on the rate of increase in SMI premium rates. This was done to prevent rises in SMI premiums from out-pacing cash benefit increases and thus excessively burdening the beneficiaries. Because of this limit, beneficiary premiums fell from 50 percent of the total cost of SMI to 25 percent. Legislation passed in 1982 has prevented, for the time being, a further increase in the percentage of premiums paid by taxpayers.

From 1972 to 1981, there was a gradual but not very stringent administrative tightening of Medicare rules that reduced to some extent the rate of growth of costs. However, estimates of program expenditures indicated an increasing gap between those costs and the revenue to pay hospital bills. This contrasted with large increases in general revenue support for SMI. Greatly increased control of all hospital costs was sought by the Carter administration through enabling legislation, but Congress would not accede to these constraints.

The Omnibus Reconciliation Act of 1981 increased the Medicare HI deductible to a level more than 12 percent higher than that scheduled under the automatic adjustment procedure set by previous legislation.[7] This change reduced budget costs by approximately $360 million in 1984.[8]

The Tax Equity and Financial Responsibility Act of 1982 (TEFRA) was the only federal legislative activity designed to reduce Medicare costs since the 1972 actions. This law profoundly changed Medicare's hospital reimbursement methods.[9] First, the basis of reimbursement was shifted from an implicit per diem system to an explicit per case system; second, case mix was incorporated into the payment system; and third, a limit was placed on the rate of allowable increase in costs per case. While reimbursement continued to be based on reasonable costs, the application of this concept was radically altered. Costs per case which were higher than 120 percent of the average (adjusted for wages and case mix for comparable hospitals), or which rose by more than the target rate over the past year, were no longer considered reasonable. TEFRA also required that the Secretary of the Department of Health and Human Services develop a prospective payment system.

The 1983 Social Security legislation included the substitution of a hospital prospective payment system for the former reasonable cost basis of reimbursement. This action represents the largest change in reimbursement policy since the establishment of Medicare. Significantly the cost-control aspect of this policy focuses on hospitals, not beneficiaries. The 1983 legislation only applies to the Medicare program. Thus, despite limits on Medicare payments, hospitals would have the opportunity to earn additional revenue from non-Medicare patients. This opportunity for cost shifting enables the hospitals to offset losses in revenue resulting from treating Medicare patients. However, those favoring controls on all hospital costs included in the law a provision through which states could obtain waivers from the basic Medicare prospective payment plan if they instituted a prospective payment proposal that covered all hospital patients.

Since the new system is applied on a per case basis, it generally results in the same payment regardless of the length of stay or the volume of services provided. This should result in lessened incentives toward volume increases. However, changes in the patient care mix may result in more complex DRGs with higher payment rates.

The Diagnostic-Related Group Prospective Payment System

The basic features of the Medicare prospective payment system are: (1) all patients are classfied into one of 468 diagnosis-related groups (DRGs); (2) with few exceptions, the hospital receives a fixed payment per DRG to cover operating costs; (3) the payment per DRG received by a hospital is a function of area wages, whether the facility is located in a rural or urban area, and the number of full-time interns and residents on its staff; and (4) capital costs and direct education are included, but the secretary of HHS is to report to Congress on methods of including these costs in the prospective rates. There is a three-year phase-in period during which the payment rates shift from being essentially based on retrospective reimbursement to being set on a national basis with adjustments based on region, staff size, and local wage rates. Thus, by 1987, reimbursement to an individual hospital to pay for the operating costs of producing services to Medicare beneficiaries will be fully based on a national prospective payment system.

One effect of a national payment rate for hospitals is to reallocate Medicare payments from relatively high-cost hospitals to those that are relatively low-cost. The majority of the savings from the prospective payment system come from the overall limit on the rate of growth of the average payment rate, not from the establishment of a national rate itself.

The current law explicitly determines how payment rates should be increased. Basically, payment rates on the average are to increase by the "market basket plus one." The market basket is a measure of the rate of increase in the prices that hospitals have to pay for their inputs, and the additional one percentage point (the intensity factor) is to provide some room for "technological change." Since the market basket price index has consistently increased more than the overall consumer price index, the new law insures that the payment rate for a Medicare illness episode will continue to increase at a faster rate than that of goods and services in general.

However, the allowed rate of increase in payments is below past growth rates and there is uncertainty among health economists as to whether this reduction in Medicare price increases can be obtained. Moreover, the rate paid by Medicare is influenced by cost-containment efforts in the private sector. If the latter does not implement complementary cost-containment policies, than the gap between public and private payment rates may become large.

The current law gives some incentive for states to implement all-payer hospital state rate-setting programs. These are programs whereby a state regulatory agency establishes mechanisms for setting hospital rates which apply to all hospitalized patients. It seems likely that the new Medicare law will result in a number of states implementing all-payer hospital rates. Some private insurers, for example, are concerned that the new Medicare law will result in cost shifts harmful to them, and they would, therefore, prefer to limit the hospital's ability to shift costs. In addition, some hospital administrators may believe that they will have more control over their fiscal situation under a state rate-setting system than under the Medicare DRG system. A state rate-setting system, with its built-in appeals process, is more likely to be sensitive to the particular needs of individual hospitals. Finally, such a system can provide a social mechanism for dealing with the growing problem of uncompensated care and can moderate a trend towards a dual medical system with one level of care for publicly financed patients and a lower quality of care for the indigent.

The probable effects of the Medicare prospective payment system are:[10]

1. There will be incentives to decrease the services provided to patients. There will likely be major disagreements about whether these reductions are an appropriate response to newly imposed constraints or represent a decline in the quality of service.[11] In addition, some hospitals will eliminate some services completely and will no longer treat certain conditions that either require services that have been dropped or that are too expensive to treat in comparison with expected payments.

2. Lengths of stay for particular diagnoses should decrease because the hospitals get no additional revenue for long stays as compared to short stays, but use of home health agencies, nursing home beds, and rehabilitation centers will likely increase. It is possible that patients receiving services in these latter settings will have more severe conditions and thus be more costly on the average than those treated before the implementation of the DRG system. There is some evidence that the decline in length of stay has already occurred. The average length of stay of Medicare patients in hospitals fell from 9.5 days in 1983, to 7.5 days in 1984.[12]

3. The number of admissions and readmissions will likely increase. Some patients who could be treated as outpatients may be treated as inpatients. In addition, there will be some incentive to space treatments or operations (if possible) rather than to do all of them during the same hospital episode since the hospital will be reimbursed for each admission.

4. Preadmission testing should increase, as it will occasionally be possible through unbundling to charge for it under Part B and collect the full DRG rate under Part A of Medicare. The law makes it illegal to unbundle services while the patient is hospitalized, but does not include outpatient services under this prohibition. If Parts A and B of Medicare were merged, it would remove existing incentives for the unbundling of what are now hospital-based services.

5. Since every DRG represents a collection of different diagnoses and conditions along with their associated treatments, it is possible that some providers may attempt to admit only certain patients within a particular DRG. Thus, the hospital may try to select only the patients who are not relatively costly to treat within a given DRG and send the sicker patients to another facility.

6. Services that have been cross-subsidized by other services are likely to be reduced since the DRG system does not include reimbursement for the former. Thus, programs in social services, nutritional counseling, health promotion, and prevention may be curtailed because, while they contribute to a decrease in the cost of posthospital care, they cause increases in inpatient costs.

Provider review organizations (PROs) will have a potentially important role in quality assurance under a DRG-based prospective payment system.[13] This is because the incentives to reduce services are much stronger in a DRG-oriented system than with traditional cost-based reimbursement.

Medicare projects a $68 billion saving over the next three years as a result of the prospective payment system.[14] While that may only postpone the insolvency of the trust fund by one year (see tables 4–3 and 4–4), $68 billion is still a substantial savings.

However, the proposal to establish uniform national DRG prices by 1987 will produce no net savings to the trust fund whatsoever.[15] For every hospital or group of hospitals that is penalized by the establishment of a single national standard, there is a corresponding hospital or group of hospitals that receives a financial gain. Since no system of price setting can ever be ideal, one can argue that the most sensible policy is to base at least some percentage of a hospital's rates on its historic cost patterns. For example, in New Jersey, a relatively complex formula has produced a pattern in which each hospital's rate for any given DRG is based roughly 50 percent on a uniform standard and roughly 50 percent on the hospital's own historical cost experience.

As for the concern that hospitals may react to the DRG system by increasing admission rates, researchers have shown that admission rates for a few surgical procedures, such as hysterectomy, vary extensively among hospital market areas, probably because of differences in physicians' practice styles. In order to determine whether such variations occur for most causes of admission, all nonobstetrical medical and surgical hospitalizations in Maine for the years 1980 to 1982 were classifed into DRGs and the variation in admission rates among thirty hospital market areas was measured. Hysterectomy rates varied 3.5 times, but 90 percent of medical and surgical admissions were in DRGs for which admission rates were even more variable, suggesting that professional discretion plays an important part in determining the rate of hospitalization for most DRGs.

Losses in hospital revenues resulting from the DRG payment system could be offset if physicians altered their admission policies to produce more income and they could still be within the limits of medical practice standards. If this type of provider behavior occurred generally, the net effect of a DRG program would be to worsen hospital cost inflation.[16] Thus, in order to be successful, cost-containment programs based on fixed, preadmission hospital rates will need to ensure effective control of hospital utilization.

The Current Method of Paying Physicians

With few exceptions, Medicare uses the customary-prevailing-reasonable (CPR) charge method to determine how much it will pay for each service provided by a physician.[17] About six thousand different services are identified and payment for each is determined by comparing the amount of physician charges with both physician and area-specific ceilings for that service.

On each claim, physicians have the option of accepting or rejecting assignment of the benefit due. Accepting Medicare assignment limits how much the physician can charge the beneficiary in exchange for a federal guarantee to pay part of the bill. Rejecting assignment allows the physician to charge the beneficiary as much as he wants, but Medicare does not guarantee collection of the billed amount.

As mentioned previously, the 1972 Social Security amendments included a provision to limit the growth in community-wide prevailing charges to a rate determined by an economic index that reflects national increases in incomes and physician-practice costs. In spite of this index, Medicare's payments for physician services have grown faster than its payments for hospital services. (See table 4–2.) The share of Medicare's total spending for personal health care allocated to physician services increased from 21.4 percent in 1975 to 22.4 percent in 1982. Although much smaller than hospital care's 1982 share of 71.3 percent, payments for physician services are considerable.

Not only is the Medicare reimbursement method for physicians unable to slow rising Medicare costs, it is hard for both patients and physicians to understand. Most of the difficulty stems from two interrelated parts of the payment method: physician billing options and beneficiary cost sharing. Frequently neither the beneficiary nor providers knows ahead of time how much Medicare will pay. Patients do not know what their cost sharing will be since, after a $75 deductible, it is 20 percent of an unknown amount on assigned claims, plus the difference between that amount and the billed charge on non-assigned claims. Moreover, physicians are unaware of how much cost sharing

Table 4–2
Medicare's Spending for Hospital Care and Physician Services: Amounts and Rates of Growth, 1975–1982

| | Annual Spending | | | |
| | Hospital Care | | Physician Services | |
Year	Dollars (billions)	Percent of Total Medicare Spending	Dollars (billions)	Percent of Total Medicare Spending
1975	11.6	74.4	3.3	21.4
1979	21.7	73.8	6.4	21.8
1980	26.0	72.8	7.8	21.8
1981	31.0	72.0	9.7	22.3
1982	3.0	71.3	11.4	22.4

| | Compound Rate of Growth (percent per year) | |
Years	Hospital Care	Physician Services
1979–82	17.2	19.2
1975–82	16.3	17.7

Source: Robert Gibson, "National Health Expenditures, 1979," *Health Care Financing Review* 2, no. 1 (Summer 1980):29–32; Robert Gibson, Daniel Waldo, and Katherine Levit, "National Health Expenditures, 1982," *Health Care Financing Review* 5, no. 1 (Fall 1983):13–15.

to bill beneficiaries on assigned claims, and they are unable to determine the probability of being paid on nonassigned claims.[18]

Another criticism of physician payment under Medicare is that it provides little incentive for physicians to utilize cost-effective treatment methods. First, as a fee-for-service system, it provides an incentive to provide more rather than fewer services. Second, CPR-determined fees for procedures do not decline as the costs of providing those services fall over time due to technological change. Third, the CPR system is biased in favor of complex treatment utilizing, for example, specialist services, as opposed to less costly primary care services.

Proposals to Change How Medicare Determines Rates of Payment

The optimal physician payment system is one that simultaneously slows the rate of growth of payments, is easy to implement and administer, is understandable by both physician and beneficiary, maintains quality and access to care, and provides an incentive to providers to offer an effective and efficient combination of services.

Is there are any one payment system that satisfies these ideals? In a practical sense, no. If fiscal pressures require that Medicare spend less for physician services, then any changes made to realize that objective will result in reductions in access to care and/or the quality of that care.

The best strategy may be a fee-for-service system combined with a prospective fee schedule.[19] Fee-for-service with a predetermined fee schedule is able to generate the information necessary to monitor the quality of and access to care, is easy to implement, and is probably relatively inexpensive to administer. Although freezing existing fees will not create an ideal fee schedule, it may be a good starting point for making judgments about the relation between fees for a specific service and costs to the provider as well as benefit to patients.

Another alternative method of determining payment rate is a fee freeze. While simple to put into effect, it would mean that some services would be overpriced relative to costs and benefits, while others would be underpriced.

Physician fee differences could also be eliminated simply by having the same fees apply to all physicians within a geographic area. Variations in rates across locales should reflect differences in the underlying nonphysician costs of providing services, such as office rentals, utility rates, and wages for employees of physicians' practices. With improvements in technology and accumulated experience, the costs of providing a particular service may fall over time, and fee schedules within particular regions should reflect this decline.

Indemnity Schedules

Some health economists support the idea of indemnity insurance. Indemnity insurance reimburses the insured beneficiary a fixed amount for a covered service. There are three advantages of the indemnity approach:[20]

1. It rewards Medicare patients for seeking care from physicians who charge relatively lower fees, since the patients would keep the difference between the indemnity amount and the physician's charge.
2. It does not eliminate price competition among physicians trying to attract Medicare patients.
3. It leaves physicians free to charge fees consistent with changes in their practice costs, market conditions, and technology.

An indemnity schedule, like a fee schedule, could incorporate relative values to reflect Medicare's assessment of the comparative costs and benefits of alternative services. Moreover, like a fee schedule, it would eliminate uncertainty over the magnitude of Medicare reimbursement levels. Physicians would be required to reveal both their fees and Medicare's indemnity amounts for the specific treatments provided. Indemnity amounts could be varied to reflect regional and community differences in living costs in order that the real value of the indemnity to the beneficiary would be uniform across the nation.

Proposals to Change Practice Arrangements

Except in the preferred provider organization (PPO), bearing financial risk typically means that the physician receives a bonus for keeping utilization and expenditures below some target figure, but is penalized financially if that figure is exceeded. For HMOs and IPAs, the target is, in effect, the premium or capitation income of the plan. If expenditures exceed plan revenues, then all physicians may lose some income; over-prescribing physicians may be penalized or dropped if the plan is to continue operating. Such organizations, especially HMOs, can also compensate physicians on a salaried basis which further reduces the incentive to provide care.[21] HMOs can also impose various types of utilization controls to influence how much care physicians provide. These are especially important as group size increases. (See chapter 7.)

PPOs differ from these plans in that they do not generally rely on targets, bonuses, and penalties to control utilization. In one version, a nonprovider organization (such as an insurer, employer, or union) negotiates fee discounts from physicians in exchange for the promise of additional patients. (See chapter

7.) Alternatively, physicians may form a PPO and market their lower fees to patient groups, who have an incentive to use the discounting physicians since it costs them more out-of-pocket if they go to a nonpreferred provider. Thus, PPOs are similar to other plans in requiring a new organizational arrangement and in limiting beneficiary choice in choosing providers, but are otherwise similar to fee-for-service, although with reduced fees.

The area-wide fiscal incentive approach differs from the other strategies in this group by setting targets for Medicare spending for all services in a geographic area, comparing actual with target spending, and then penalizing or rewarding all physicians in an area depending on whether the locale experienced a deficit (with actual spending exceeding the target), or a surplus (with spending below the target). In effect, this proposal would place financial liability for managing services in an area on all physicians, and would leave the method of achieving fiscal control up to the physicians themselves. Unlike other plans, area-wide incentives would not directly limit beneficiary freedom in choosing providers, although there could be interarea disincentives that would directly limit access.[22]

There are various reasons why none of these proposals is reasonable as the optimal approach for paying physicians under Medicare. First, physicians and beneficiaries would have to be forced to form or join such alternative systems; and organizing these new arrangements would present major problems. Second, the estimates of cost savings are usually based on isolated studies, most of which involve atypical participants. These estimates undoubtedly exaggerate total cost savings if these plans were made compulsory.

Moreover, none of these proposals offers a good mechanism for deciding how much Medicare should pay for care of a given quality. In the short run, the pressure to cut costs might lead to an administrative decision irrespective of specific organizational arrangements such as "95 percent of what was paid last year." However, over time, Medicare would still have to determine capitation rates as well as individual or area budget targets. Medicare's difficulty in determining an appropriate capitation rate for enrolling beneficiaries in existing HMOs is a good example of the problems which occur. (See chapter 7.)

In spite of these difficulties, Medicare should continue to encourage the development of new practice arrangements as competing alternatives to, although not as complete substitutes for, fee-for-service practice. Both Medicare and private sector initiatives—such as HMOs, PPOs, and IPAs—are likely to increase pressure on fee-for-service practitioners to restrain the rate of growth of fees and expenditures. Even in the absence of change in the CPR system, competition-induced reductions in the growth of fees would produce savings for the Medicare programs. Simultaneously, competition among alternative delivery systems would likely assure beneficiaries more protection against poor quality and limited access than would a government-sanctioned monopoly system.[23]

Some recent proposals would change what Medicare pays for rather than reimbursing for particular items of service provided. These reforms would have Medicare pay for packages of services. One suggestion would combine payment to the provider (on behalf of an inpatient) with the reimbursement to the hospital based on the patient's DRG.

Another proposal would collapse sets of detailed medical procedures and services into smaller but more comprehensive groups. For example, all types of office visits, regardless of length or complexity, would comprise one group, all hospital visits another group, and all laboratory tests a third. These groupings of services would still be reimbursed on a fee-for-service basis, but physicians could not increase billings by unbundling (that is, disaggregating) services from the overall package.

There is little or no experience with paying physicians on a per diagnosis, per episode of illness, or per grouped service-package basis. The unfamiliarity with defining, measuring, and constructing diagnosis-related groups or episodes of illness for ambulatory care and physician services is a major disadvantage of adopting these proposals as short-run solutions to Medicare's cost problems.

Medicare Financing

Revenues for the support of HI come primarily from a portion of the Social Security payroll tax. Employers and employees covered by the program each contribute 1.3 percent of earnings up to a maximum level (in 1984, the first $37,800 of earnings), with the rate scheduled to increase to 1.35 percent in 1985, and 1.45 percent in 1986. Under current law, general revenues cannot be used to make up any shortfall between outlays required to pay benefits and the balance in the trust fund.[24]

In contrast, SMI revenues are obtained from premiums and general revenues. The premium amount (in 1985, $15.50 per month) is increased by law every year, with a contribution from general revenues making up the difference between premium income and outlays. In fiscal year 1983, general revenues required to meet this difference totaled about $14 billion, or 77 percent of SMI funding.[25]

The Medicare program will encounter serious funding problems in the near future. Under current policies, the HI trust fund will be entirely depleted around 1989 or 1990, while required contributions from general revenues to support physician benefits will continue to grow at a much more rapid rate than the growth in general revenues. The basic problem is that spending on medical care is growing much more rapidly than national income, with demographic trends such as the aging of the population explaining only a small part of the difference. Moreover, because of the projected 1986 federal budget deficit of more than $200 billion, the amount of additional financial resources that might be allocated to Medicare is severely limited.

HI Financing

Under present policies, depletion of the HI trust fund will occur within five years. (See table 4–3.) The end-of-year balances are projected to decline after 1987, as annual outlays exceed annual income by increasing amounts. By 1995, the annual deficit is expected to be more than $60 billion, or more than one-third of the projected expenditures, and the negative trust fund balance will exceed $250 billion.

However, under the DRG program in which payments per admission were increased by only one percentage point more than the rate of increase of hospital input prices, the projected depletion date would be three years later (1992). (See table 4–4.) The projected deficits would still grow larger each year, even under this restricted growth in outlays. By 1995 the annual deficit would be about $30 billion and the negative balance over $90 billion.

From 1985 to 1995, Medicare outlays are projected to grow at a 12.4 percent annual rate, while revenues are projected to increase at a 7.9 percent rate. This increase reflects the influences of general inflation, growth in the

Table 4–3
Baseline Projections of Hospital Insurance Trust Fund Outlays, Income, and Balances
(by calendar year, in billions of dollars)

Year	Outlays	Income	Annual Surplus (Excluding Any Negative Interest)	Year-end Balance
1981	30.7	35.7	5.0	18.8
1982	36.1	25.6	− 10.6	8.2
1983	40.6	43.8	3.1	11.3
1984	46.5	46.3	− 0.2	11.1
1985	51.2	53.4	2.2	13.3
1986	57.3	66.4	9.1	22.4
1987	64.5	66.7	2.2	24.6
1988	72.5	66.8	− 5.7	18.9
1989	81.5	70.7	− 10.8	8.1
1990	91.7	74.5	− 17.2	− 9.1
1991	103.1	77.9	− 25.2	− 34.3
1992	115.8	81.1	− 34.7	− 69.0
1993	130.1	83.9	− 46.2	− 115.2
1994	146.2	86.3	− 59.9	− 175.1
1995	164.5	87.7	− 76.8	− 251.9

Source: Congressional Budget Office estimates based on February 1983 budget and economic assumptions, but updated to reflect the Social Security amendments of 1983 (P.L. 98-21).

Table 4–4
Projections of Hospital Insurance Trust Fund Outlays, Income, and Balances
under Assumption of More Stringent DRG Rates after 1985ᵃ
(by calendar year, in billions of dollars)

Year	Outlays	Income	Annual Surplus (Excluding Any Negative Interest)	Year-end Balance
1986	57.3	66.4	9.1	22.4
1987	62.1	66.9	4.8	27.2
1988	68.3	67.1	− 1.2	26.0
1989	75.1	71.5	− 3.6	22.4
1990	82.6	75.9	− 6.7	15.7
1991	90.9	80.1	− 10.8	4.9
1992	99.9	84.6	− 15.3	− 10.4
1993	109.8	89.1	− 20.7	− 31.1
1994	120.8	93.6	− 27.2	− 58.3
1995	133.0	98.0	− 35.0	− 93.3

Source: Congressional Budget Office estimates based on February 1983 budget and economic assumptions, but updated to reflect the Social Security amendments of 1983 (P.L. 98-21).
ᵃAssumes diagnosis-related group (DRG) rates are increased one percentage point per year faster than the increase in the hospital market basket.

eligible population and its aging, and changes in the nature of hospital care. General inflation accounts for a significant portion of the increase in hospital costs, but does not itself contribute to the financing problem since it is also reflected in revenue growth. Over the ten-year period, the GNP deflator is projected to increase at a 3.8 percent annual rate. The overall rate of increase in hospital input prices is projected to grow somewhat faster at an annual rate of 5.7 percent.

Changes in the age composition of the population are projected to account for 2.2 percentage points of the growth in HI outlays. Of this, 1.9 percentage points reflect growth in the number of enrollees, while 0.25 percentage points are caused by the expected aging of the elderly population. While HI claims increase with age, the aging of the Medicare population is sufficiently gradual to not be a major contributor to expenditure growth during this period. Real outlays per enrollee are expected to grow at slightly more than 4 percent per year after 1985. This figure reflects both the impact of a higher admission rate per Medicare enrollee and a higher expense per hospital stay.

SMI Financing

Between 1978 and 1982, total SMI benefits rose at an annual rate of 21 percent. About one-tenth of this growth was caused by expansion in the enrolled population, and the remainder to a combination of increases in prices and utilization of services.

Although it is difficult to separate the price and quantity factors, changes in the latter are particularly important in SMI, accounting for almost half of total per capita growth in outlays. For example, total per capita physicians services—which constitute over 72 percent of SMI benefits—grew at an annual rate of 18 percent during the period 1978–1982.[26]

Problems raised by the rapid growth expected in SMI are closely related to concern over the size of the federal budget deficit, which is expected to be over $200 billion in 1985. Since by law, appropriations from general revenues to SMI must be sufficient to guarantee solvency of the trust fund, SMI does not face a major crisis in financing per se. Rather, concern arises over this part of Medicare because the projected growth of SMI is far higher than the increase in general revenues.

Like HI, outlays under SMI are projected to increase rapidly, by almost 16 percent per year through 1988. To finance this increase, general revenue contributions must rise even faster, averaging about 17 percent per year. Thus, the proportion of general revenues necessary to finance the SMI trust fund is expected to rise from 3.7 percent to 5.7 percent between 1982 and 1988. If the share of general revenues contributed to the SMI trust fund were not permitted to increase, expenditures would have to be reduced or premiums increased by almost $27 billion from 1984 to 1988, which represents about 19 percent of all SMI expenditures for that period.[27]

If both revenues and SMI outlays were to continue growing at the same annual rates now projected through 1988, SMI would require a transfer of more than 11 percent of general revenues not allocated to other purposes in 1995. Alternatively, even if SMI outlays only rose at an annual rate of 12 percent and general revenues rose by 8 percent annually, the share of such revenues necessary to fund SMI would still rise to more than 7 percent in 1995.

Medicare Financing Policy Options

The problems facing Medicare are essentially threefold: the number of beneficiaries is rising, the volume of services per beneficiary is growing, and the unit costs of those services to the federal government are increasing. Unless policy options consider these underlying problems, the Medicare program likely will remain in financial difficulty.

There are four possible approaches to reducing Medicare's financial problems:

1. reduce the number of persons covered,
2. reduce the number of services included in the program,

3. pay less for each covered service, and
4. increase the proportion of costs paid by the elderly or taxpayers as a whole.

Restrict Coverage

Expenditures could be reduced by either raising the initial age of eligibility or by excluding some persons from the program. The major argument for raising the age of eligibility is that 65 year-olds are presently in better health than when the program started in 1966, and thus have less need for Medicare. However, older persons continue to retire earlier, so there would be a drop in health care coverage if the age of eligibility were increased. Moreover, for those not retiring at age 65, Medicare presently pays a low percentage of health care costs, since recent legislation has made Medicare secondary to employer-provided coverage. This Medicare coverage could be coupled with increases in the retirement age under Social Security.

A more controversial proposal is to eliminate the eligibility of some persons, for example, those with high incomes. While this exclusion would permit either higher benefits or lower taxes for some, it would represent a major change in the philosophy of the program. Many of those who consider varying the premium levels or relating cost sharing to the income of the beneficiaries, object to eliminating coverage for any of the elderly population.

Pay for Fewer Services

The number of services paid for could be reduced either through direct limitations or through incentives to beneficiaries and/or providers. Direct controls could, for example, involve decisions not to pay for certain health services. Currently, rules concerning what procedures are covered are made by Medicare or its intermediaries. For example, reimbursements may be restricted on the basis of where treatment was obtained or the relevance of that treatment to a particular diagnosis. Additional limitations on coverage could include cost restrictions or restraints on the use of complex procedures. Peer review organizations (PROs) could refuse payment for courses of treatment that differ from local medical norms, although the strictness with which these controls were implemented could be highly controversial. The Medicare program presently has a number of indirect incentives to control use of services. These include cost sharing and, more recently, the new hospital prospective payment system based on DRGs. Medicare does require some beneficiary cost sharing, particularly for physician and outpatient services. While this may limit utilization, the degree of actual cost sharing is relatively low due to the extensive purchase of supplemental insurance. About 70 percent of Medicare beneficiaries are covered either by Medicaid or by a private supplemental insurance policy.

The new DRG hospital payment system also gives hospitals the incentive to be more efficient in the treatment of each case, and will probably reduce the number of services provided during each hospital stay. However, as indicated previously, it will also encourage additional hospital admissions, and the DRG system does not improve incentives to provide optimal hospital care. For example, the DRG system provides no economic incentive to discourage choice of a more expensive surgical treatment instead of an alternative treatment with lower costs that is classified within a different DRG. Thus, even this major change in hospital reimbursement policy under Medicare does not necessarily lead one to the most cost-effective care.

In contrast to incentives for providers, additional cost sharing could reduce the volume of services by raising the net price to the patient. While there is little evidence on the effects of cost sharing on utilization by Medicare beneficiaries, numerous studies of those persons under age 65 (and therefore not covered by Medicare) indicate utilization declines as cost sharing rises. However, given the widespread coverage of private supplemental insurance, increased cost sharing under Medicare would largely shift costs to the beneficiaries and those paying the supplemental insurance premiums (for example, former employers), but would have minimal impact on the volume of services.

Pay Less for Each Service

Although reducing reimbursements for each unit of service provided can produce considerable short-run savings, this policy does not directly focus on the basic factors causing higher Medicare costs. Indeed, lower reimbursements may cause providers to increase services to maintain income, thereby offsetting some government savings. For example, cuts in physician reimbursement appear to have increased billings.[28]

Reduced access to services by Medicare beneficiaries is a real possibility if the level of reimbursements is severely reduced. When providers are required to accept Medicare reimbursements as payment in full, as with hospital care, some providers may find they no longer want to serve Medicare patients at the prevailing rates. Moreover, providers continuing to serve Medicare beneficiaries may end up delivering a lower quality of care. When assignment is voluntary providers may seek amounts above Medicare's rates from beneficiaries. In this situation physicians generally react to a decline in government reimbursements by increasing the amounts obtained from their patients. Alternatively, they may refuse to treat those elderly patients who cannot afford to pay a higher proportion of the bill than they previously would have paid.

Shift Responsibility to Beneficiaries or Taxpayers

Medicare beneficiaries could pay a greater proportion of health care costs through overall increases in premiums, premium increases limited to higher-income beneficiaries, or higher coinsurance rates for the users of such care. Revenues for Medicare could be increased from the payroll and general tax sources that are presently used to finance the system or by changing the way in which revenue is obtained.

Overall premium increases would spread the burden among the largest number of individuals, while relating cost sharing to utilization of services would have more of an impact on beneficiaries' incentives for use of care.

Placing higher premiums for SMI into effect or introducing an HI premium for the first time would have an effect similar to a tax increase. That is, they would increase revenues to fund Medicare outlays, without necessarily changing the structure or nature of the program. However, with such policies, the burden would fall on a different group of persons than would be the case with a general tax increase. For purposes of equity, premiums could be related to income so that the major increases in premiums were absorbed by the high-income elderly.

Raising coinsurance rates would shift costs to beneficiaries and reduce utilization. But the expansion of private supplemental insurance to Medicare would mean that some persons could eliminate cost sharing altogether. These individuals would still pay a higher percentage of total cost than before because of higher insurance premiums. However, they would not have an incentive to use fewer services.

A Medicare Voucher System

An alternative approach to the Medicare financing problem is a voucher system. Rather than covering the cost of health care regardless of its efficiency, as is the case with health insurance and the current Medicare and Medicaid programs, the voucher system would be established at a level that would essentially only cover the cost of an efficient health care plan. If a consumer wished to enroll in a less efficient or more expensive plan, he would pay the entire additional cost of coverage. The vouchers could be provided by employers instead of their current health benefit systems, or they could be paid for by governments, replacing the current Medicare and Medicaid systems. It is anticipated that the competition resulting from a voucher system would assist in reducing the rate of growth in medical care expenditures.

Vouchers offer several advantages from the perspective of the federal government. Currently, Medicaid and Medicare expenditures are not directly controllable so that price and utilization increases directly raise budgetary outlays. Vouchers would put an upper limit on annual government obligations, with the only variable factor being the number of persons eligible for services. Another advantage is that a voucher system would greatly reduce the government's role in increasing medical care costs. Once the monetary value of the voucher has been determined, the government would only need to monitor market operations to assure reasonable business practice; it would no longer be in a potentially adversarial role with providers.[29]

Problems of Adverse Selection

The major problem with a voucher system is adverse selection.[30] Adverse selection occurs when people who are above-average users of medical care are concentrated in certain health care plans. This causes premiums to reflect not only differences in plan efficiency but also variations in enrollee mix.

In theory, establishing premiums and vouchers according to risk classifications (health status) is an attractive solution to the adverse selection problem, but it may be impractical partly due to the difficulty of accurately measuring health status. Unless the adverse selection issue is solved, some carriers would have incentives to attract potential enrollees whose expected utilization is less than that indicated by their risk category.

Adverse selection is likely to be an even bigger difficulty in a voluntary plan in which people have the option of remaining in the existing Medicare plan. The basic Medicare plan could end up with all the high-cost enrollees because low-risk beneficiaries would be more likely to join low-option plans.

A mandatory voucher system does not eliminate the problem of adverse selection. It merely transfers the risk from the federal government to the private sector. If the private carriers believe that the risk adjustments are not adequate, they will be unlikely to participate in the program. If substantial adverse selection occurs and cannot be controlled, a voucher system will be unworkable.

Advocates of vouchers seem not to appreciate the amount of consumer education necessary in regard to health plan alternatives which must be provided to assure both reasonable choice and consumer protection. As delivery and payment systems have evolved from conventional insurance plans to preferred provider organizations, HMOs, and other alternative systems, the structure and performance of the health delivery system has become more complex. This makes it more difficult for consumers to understand even in the absence of vouchers.

Implementation Costs

A voucher plan would eliminate the government's ability to command below-market prices that is presently enjoys because Medicare is such a large purchaser of medical care. While the government does not have unlimited monopoly power, a voucher system would probably result in a 10 to 20 percent increase in hospital charges for Medicare beneficiaries. Start-up costs of the system and the regulatory structure would also have to be included in the budget. This implies that not only would it be several years before any savings might result from the voucher system, but also that the cost to Medicare might increase substantially in the meantime.

In order to determine whether adverse selection would be a major problem, demonstration and evaluation projects would need to be undertaken. Such projects also might help to decide whether or not alternative health plans can attract enrollees and whether the administration and regulation of a voucher plan is really feasible.

Medigap Insurance

Because Medicare has covered a declining fraction of the health insurance costs of the elderly over time, many persons covered by Medicare purchase supplementary insurance. This insurance is commonly known as Medigap insurance, because it is designed to eliminate some of the gaps in coverage under Medicare.

The existence of Medigap insurance causes several problems. First, the private supplemental policies vary considerably, often making it difficult for people to understand their provisions. It is even believed that some elderly people have unnecessary or duplicate policies. For example, the National Medical Care Utilization and Expenditure Survey, undertaken in 1980, found that 17 percent of aged Medicare enrollees had two or more private health insurance policies.[31]

Second, since about two-thirds of all Medicare beneficiaries buy supplementary (Medigap) insurance to protect themselves financially against the deductible and coinsurance provisions of Medicare, supplementary health insurance (which has a high loading charge), probably contributes to the misallocation of health care resources by discouraging patients and their physicians from obtaining less costly but equally effective forms of treatment.[32]

Third, Medigap policies generally add to the paperwork the elderly need to deal with in order to be reimbursed. Unless there is an agreement that the Medicare fiscal agent directly passes on processed claims to the Medigap insurer, the beneficiary must apply for reimbursement first to Medicare and subsequently to the private insurer.

Finally, the premiums for Medigap policies are rising and for some elderly persons are so expensive as to make such insurance unaffordable. The rising costs of Medigap policies are illustrated by recent actions of Maryland Blue Cross-Blue Shield. In the first plan, the "65 program," monthly premiums of $14.80 in 1981 were increased to $19.20 in 1982, resulting in an annual premium of $230.40. This plan covers most of Medicare's Part A cost sharing but not all of Part B cost sharing. Neither the Part B deductible nor Part B coinsurance for office visits are covered. In the second plan, "preferred

Medicare supplemental insurance," monthly premiums were $33.74 in 1981, rose to $50.20 in 1982, for an annual total of $602.40, and reached $675.84 per year in 1983. This Medigap option covers all cost sharing under Medicare, includes drug costs after a $3 deductible per prescription, and provides up to 365 days of hospital care per benefit period.[33]

Nursing Care

Medicare is a minor factor in the nursing home market. The program provides only 2 percent of total industry revenues, and over half the facilities certified for Medicare (two-thirds of all skilled facilities) reported fewer than 5 percent Medicare patient days in 1977. In contrast, Medicaid provides half the industry's revenues while supporting, at least to some degree, three-fifths of nursing home residents.[34] Medicare benefits are basically limited to short-term nursing home care. Thus, in 1977, Medicare-covered stays averaged 28.1 days compared with a 227-day average stay for all patients in skilled nursing homes.[35]

Nursing home provision of Medicare-covered days per beneficiary dropped 17 percent between 1977 and 1979, with no change in eligibility or perceived decline in the demand for service.[36] One result has been extended hospital stays while patients search for a nursing home willing to admit them. Estimates of these so-called "back-up days" range from 1 million to 9.2 million per year. Medicare pays for most of these back-up days in the hospital, where routine costs are about four times greater than they would be in a nursing home. Limited access to nursing homes also imposes costs on the beneficiaries themselves and state Medicaid programs. When admitted to a nursing home, patients (or Medicaid, for patients who qualify) pay for services that Medicare could cover.

The difference in the Medicare and Medicaid role in nursing home activities results from differences in their definitions of covered care. First, Medicare covers skilled care while Medicaid reimburses for skilled and intermediate care. Second, Medicare defines skilled care much more narrowly than do many state Medicaid programs.

Designed by law as an alternative to extended hospital stays, the Medicare skilled nursing home benefit offers elderly and disabled beneficiaries no more than 100 days of intensive nursing or rehabilitation care following a hospital stay. Most Medicare patients obtain short-term coverage for nursing or rehabilitation services delivered on a daily basis.

In contrast, Medicaid, which finances many health services for some categories of poor people, pays for relatively long nursing home stays in both skilled and intermediate care facilities. Medicaid benefits for skilled patient care are not limited to 100 days and do not require a previous hospital stay. A more important factor in explaining longer stays is the fact that in many states Medicaid patients are receiving general rather than specific skilled nursing services, including supervision of aide-delivered assistance with daily activities.

Medicare limits its coverage and liabilities for nursing homes in several ways. Medicare cannot legally cover custodial care. To assure that care is "skilled" in ambiguous cases, coverage is related to changes in the patient's condition. Medicare also limits its payment levels by determining reimbursement after care has been provided, thus, putting nursing homes at financial risk for claims that Medicare's fiscal agents (intermediaries) may reject. Because coverage is not determined until after care has been delivered (that is, when the nursing home submits a claim), to assure certainty of payment, minimize paperwork, and avoid financial uncertainty, homes are likely to inform patients not receiving treatments clearly labeled skilled that Medicare does not cover the services being rendered.

Unless patients are receiving specific treatments (such as intravenous or intramuscular injections, tube feedings, or aspiration of air passages), Medicare coverage for skilled nursing care is difficult to obtain. The law does authorize coverage for nursing observation or supervision of unskilled services, but regulations limit coverage for observation to patients whose condition is "unstable" and supervision to cases with a "high probability" of complications. It is the responsibility of the nursing home to prove that the patient actually was unstable or had a high probability of complications. A patient whose only needs are for assistance in daily living activities or whose poor health reflects the aging process and not a specific medical condition would not be eligible for Medicare coverage. Thus, because of these regulations, Medicare nursing home benefits are basically limited to short-term care.

Medicare requires more rigorous health and safety standards and greater staffing than Medicaid and may impose more burdensome accounting and record-keeping requirements. Neither of these administrative costs is likely to be fully reimbursed since Medicare reimbursements are based on the averaging of costs for both Medicare and non-Medicare patients. Partly because of these overhead costs, on a national basis, a third of Medicaid-certified nursing homes do not seek Medicare certification.

Nursing home administrators in some states are reluctant to deal with Medicare due to experiences with the program in its early years. The Medicare program began imposing rigorous claims review in 1969. The result was a 60 percent decline in Medicare-covered nursing home days between 1969 and 1972.[37] Much of the decline reflected retroactive denial of claims after care had been delivered, which has left the lasting impression that the program can easily change regulations that have a major impact on nursing home reimbursement. Without strong financial incentives, some nursing homes are unwilling to participate in Medicare.

Medicare patients' brief nursing home stay relative to Medicaid patients' also creates a demand on staff time, and makes the former less desirable as patients. In 1981, 86 percent of Medicare patients stayed in nursing homes for fewer than 60 days (including noncovered as well as covered time), while more than half the Medicaid skilled patients in skilled facilities stayed longer than 180 days.[38] New admissions require patient evaluations and development of treatment plans; discharges require preparation and training for self-care. Instead of investing this time in patients with relatively short stays, nursing homes may prefer to accept patients who will be there for a considerably longer period.

Because Medicare is a federal program, solutions to eligibility problems regarding nursing home patients require changes in federal policy. Given current benefits, the program has two options: (1) the program could consider only the federal cost problem, accepting limited access but reducing the reimbursement rates for patients "backed-up" in hospitals; or (2) the program could address all parties' problems in improving access for Medicare beneficiaries by changing many of its policies to conform to general practice among nursing homes.

Congress supported the first option with 1980 legislation that authorized payment for back-up days at average Medicaid-skilled nursing home rates.[39] However, the Department of Health and Human Services has been slow to implement this provision. The problem is that limiting payment for some hospital days does not eliminate the fixed costs of hospitalization. Moreover, while this strategy would reduce the federal government's financial burden, there would not be a commensurate decline in social costs. Lower rates for back-up days would eliminate any incentive hospitals have to retain patients that do not belong there. However, lower rates will not eliminate back-ups that simply reflect placement problems. To the extent that hospitals cannot or do not reduce the cost of these days, payers other than Medicare will bear these costs.

Another approach would be to have Medicare cut costs by reducing access barriers for Medicare patients. As a small purchaser in a large market, Medicare cannot by itself change the nursing home industry. However, the program could get more service from that industry by adjusting its policies to industry practice.

More nursing homes would probably participate in Medicare if the program allowed them to accept payment at Medicaid rates or developed its own Medicare prospective payment system. Nursing homes would probably have more Medicare patients if reimbursement rates reflected the above-average costs of intensive service and/or below-average stays for some patients. These reforms would probably do much more to eliminate hospital back-up days than lowering hospital reimbursement rates.

The Reagan Budget Proposals and Recent Changes in Medicare Charges

The Reagan administration is asking Congress for an additional one-year freeze in the Medicare payment rates for physicians. Since the Deficit Reduction Act of 1984 froze all fees for treating Medicare patients until October 1985, this additional freeze would be effective until October 1986.

Overall, the Medicare proposals are projected to reduce program outlays by about $3 billion in fiscal 1986, and possibly as much as $19 billion to $20 billion over the fiscal years 1986 to 1988, the largest single domestic program cut in the proposed 1986 budget.[40]

The rates Medicare pays hospitals for each patient admitted would be frozen at current levels for fiscal 1986 instead of being increased to cover inflation. In fiscal 1987 and 1988, they would be allowed to rise to keep pace with the inflation rate for the so-called medical market basket, an economic indicator based on the package of items that hospitals buy. The market basket increase usually runs higher than overall inflation in the economy. Projected fiscal 1986 savings would be $2.03 billion. With rates paid to doctors frozen at current levels, the projected fiscal 1986 savings would be $600 million.

The so-called "indirect" special Medicare allowance to teaching hospitals —where interns, residents, and other training personnel participate in teaching programs while performing hospital services as well—would be cut by 50 percent from the maximum rate, perhaps in fiscal 1986 or perhaps over the next three years.[41] In the indirect allowance, a hospital gets a higher rate of reimbursement if it has a large number of trainees. Projected fiscal 1986 savings for a three-year phase-in would total $250 million.

The basic premium for the Medicare program covering doctors' bills and other services rose 6 percent in 1985, from $14.60 to $15.50 a month.[42] This rate is being charged because the Social Security amendments passed in 1983 require the monthly premium to equal 25 percent of the expected average costs of the program for enrollees during 1984 and 1985. In the new budget proposals the monthly premium of participants in Part B of Medicare are expected to increase from 25 percent to 35 percent of program costs. The administration expects the savings to be $375 million in fiscal 1986. The deductible would remain at $75 in 1986 and then rise substantially in future years to keep pace with inflation.

The Senate has accepted the compromise recommendations of its budget committee with regard to President Reagan's proposals. The overall cuts in Medicare would total $18.3 billion over three years or nearly as much as the administration requested.[43]

Summary

The Medicare program finances a large share of the health care costs of older people, the disabled, and those with end-stage renal disease. Medicare costs have risen extremely rapidly since the inception of the program in 1966.

The Medicare program makes extensive use of coinsurance and deductibles. While these are intended to deter unnecessary utilization, a majority of the elderly purchase supplementary insurance which negates the cost-sharing provisions of Medicare.

Medicare has gradually increased its cost-containment policies. Since 1981, there has been an increase in cost sharing and the imposition of a prospective payment system for hospitals based on diagnostic-related groups (DRGs). The DRG system will likely result in shorter stays for most hospitalized elderly patients with some decrease in provided services. Moreover, services such as health promotion, which traditionally have been cross-subsidized, are likely to be cut back or eliminated.

The Medicare program faces major financing problems in the near future. Without major increases in revenues or decreases in expenditures, the hospital insurance (HI) trust fund will be completely depleted by 1990. Moreover, the proportion of general revenues needed to finance supplementary medical insurance (SMI) will have to increase rapidly to avoid fast rising premiums. While a number of policy options exist, given the current political climate in the United States, it is likely that the elderly will be called upon to finance an increasing share of Medicare costs.

Medicare provides little assistance to residents of nursing homes. By comparison, the Medicaid program provides some support to about 60 percent of all nursing home residents. The main reasons for the limited coverage of nursing services by Medicare are: (1) Medicare does not pay for custodial care; (2) Medicare only reimburses after care has been delivered, putting nursing homes at financial risk; and (3) the administrative burden on nursing homes in regard to documentation of services is excessive. More nursing homes would enroll in Medicare if they were reimbursed at Medicaid rates or developed its own prospective payment system.

The Reagan administration's 1986 budget reduces the federal share of support for Medicare. It limits payments to providers and increases consumer cost sharing. As of April 1985, the Senate had made only minor changes in the Reagan budget with regard to Medicare.

Notes

1. William Hsiao and Nancy Kelly, "Medicare Benefits: A Reassessment," *Milbank Memorial Fund Quarterly/Health and Society* 62, no. 2 (1984):209.

2. A.A. Scitovsky and N.M. Snyder, "Effect of Co-insurance on Use of Physicians' Services," *Social Security Bulletin* 35, no. 6 (June 1972):3–19.

3. A.A. Scitovsky and N. McCall, "Co-insurance and the Demand for Physician Services: Four Years Later," *Social Security Bulletin* 40, no. 5 (May 1977):19–27.

4. J.P. Newhouse et al., "Some Interim Results from a Controlled Trial of Cost Sharing in Health Insurance," *New England Journal of Medicine* 305, no. 25 (December 17, 1981):1501–07.

5. Hsiao and Kelly, op. cit., p. 215.

6. Hsiao and Kelly, op. cit., p. 217.

7. Stephen Long, Russell Settle, and Charles Link, "Who Bears the Burden of Medicare Cost Sharing?" *Inquiry* 19, no. 3 (Fall 1982):222.

8. J.A. Svahn, "Omnibus Reconciliation Act of 1981 Legislative History and Summary of OASDI and Medicare Provisions," *Social Security Bulletin* 44 (October 1981):3–24.

9. Judith, Lave, "Hospital Reimbursement Under Medicare," *Milbank Memorial Fund Quarterly/Health and Society* 62, no. 2 (1984):253.

10. Ibid., p. 261.

11. W. Schwartz, "The Competitive Strategy: Will It Affect the Quality of Care?" in J.A. Meyer, ed., *Market Reform in Health Care* (Washington, D.C.: American Enterprise Institute, 1983), pp. 15–21.

12. "Medicare Quick Release Criticized," *The Evening Sun* (Baltimore), February 26, 1985, p. A-9.

13. Bruce Vladeck, Comment on "Hospital Reimbursement Under Medicare," *Milbank Memorial Fund Quarterly/Health and Society* 62, no. 2 (1984):272.

14. U.S. Senate, Special Committee on Aging, *Prospects for Medicare's Hospital Insurance Trust Fund* (Washington, D.C.: U.S. Government Printing Office, 1983).

15. Vladek, op. cit., p. 270.

16. John E. Wennberg, Klim McPherson, and Philip Caper, "Will Payment on Diagnosis-Related Groups Control Hospital Costs?" *New England Journal of Medicine* 311, no. 5 (August 2, 1984):295.

17. R.R. Bovbjerg, P.J. Held, and M.V. Pauly, "Pro-competitive Health Insurance Proposals and Their Implications for Medicare's End-State Renal Disease Program," *Seminars in Nephrology* 2, no. 2 (1982):134–72.

18. Jack Hadley, "How Should Medicare Pay Physicians?" *Milbank Memorial Fund Quarterly/Health and Society* 62, no. 2 (1984):283.

19. Ibid., p. 281.

20. Ibid., p. 292.

21. P. Held and U. Reinhardt, eds., *Analysis of Economic Performance in Medical Groups,* project report no. 79–05 (Princeton: Mathematica Policy Research, 1980), p. 93.

22. Jack Hadley, Critique of Peter Fox's "Physician Reimbursement Under Medicare: An Overview and Proposal for Area-wide Physician Incentive," in U.S. House of Representatives, Committee on Ways and Means, Conference on the Future of Medicare, November 29–30, 1983.

23. Bovberg, Held, and Pauly, op. cit., pp. 134–72.

24. Paul Ginsburg and Marilyn Moon, "An Introduction to the Medicare Financing Problem," *Milbank Memorial Fund Quarterly/Health and Society* 62, no. 2 (1984):167.

25. Ibid., pp. 167–68.

26. Ibid., pp. 173–74.

27. Ibid., pp. 170–71.

28. T. Rice and N. McCall, "Changes in Medicare Reimbursement in Colorado: Impact on Physicians' Economic Behavior," *Health Care Financing Review* 3 (June 1982):67–85.

29. Harold Luft, "On the Use of Vouchers for Medicare," *Milbank Memorial Fund Quarterly/Health and Society* 62, no. 2 (1984):238.

30. Ibid., p. 239.

31. Stephen Garfinkel and Larry Corder, "The Extent of Supplemental Health Insurance Plans Among Aged Medicare Beneficiaries," in press.

32. Eli Ginzberg, Comment on "Medicare Benefits: A Reassessment," *Milbank Memorial Fund Quarterly/Health and Society* 62, no. 2 (1984):230.

33. Marian Gornick, James Beebe, and Ronald Prihoda, "Options for Change Under Medicare: Impact of a Cap on Catastrophic Illness Expense," *Health Care Financing Review* 5, no. 1 (Fall 1983):41.

34. National Center for Health Statistics, "National Nursing Home Survey." Mimeographed. Hyattsville, Md., 1977.

35. C. Helbing, "Medicare Use of Skilled Nursing Facilities, 1976–1977," Health Care Financing Notes, HEW Publication No. (HCFA)-03201 (Washington, D.C.: Health Care Financing Administration and National Center for Health Statistics, 1978), p. 18.

36. Judith Feder and William Scanlon, "The Under-used Benefit: Medicare's Coverage of Nursing Home Care," *Milbank Memorial Fund Quarterly/Health and Society* 60, no. 4 (1982):604.

37. Helbing, op. cit., p. 21.

38. Feder and Scanlon, op. cit., p. 624.

39. Ibid., p. 630.

40. Spencer Rich, "Year Freeze Eyed for Medicare Rates," *The Washington Post,* December 27, 1984, p. A-1.

41. Ibid., p. A-10.

42. "Medicare Rate Boost Set for January," *The Baltimore Sun,* September 28, 1984, p. 3-A.

43. Helen Dawar, "Reagan, Senators Agree on Package to Trim Deficit," *The Washington Post,* April 24, 1985, p. A-7.

5
Some Economic Aspects of Hospital Behavior

T his chapter focuses on ways in which the hospital sector is adapting to the changing economic environment. New methods of reimbursement, rising intensity of competition, and the growth of for-profit hospital chains are among the more important topics considered.

Hospital Statistics

Significant 1950–1983 trend data for nonfederal, short-term hospitals are presented in table 5–1. The number of beds per thousand population increased 30 percent over the thirty-three-year period, but was practically unchanged from 1975 to 1983. Inpatient admissions rose 117 percent from 1950 to 1983, but rose less than 10 percent from 1975 to 1983. The average length of stay fluctuated slightly in the period under consideration and was 7.3 percent lower in 1983 than in 1950. However, the inpatient population in absolute numbers (average daily census) has continued to rise, reaching 749,000 in 1983.

Outpatient care has been an increasingly important hospital activity. Statistics indicate a steep rise, especially in emergency room and private diagnostic services. From 1957 to 1982, oupatient visits increased from 67 million to 248 million, a gain of 270 percent. This was nearly 4 times more rapid than the growth rate for hospital admissions, and it indicates some degree of substitution of outpatient care for inpatient care.[1]

From 1982 to 1983, the number of hospital outpatient visits fell 15.3 percent, a rapid rate of decline.[2] This reflects the increased competition facing hospitals from walk-in clinics and health maintenance organizations.

Full-time personnel (or their equivalents in part-time workers) rose 368 percent from 1950 to 1983, and totaled 3.1 million in 1983. The personnel–patient ratio rose 101 percent to a 1983 high of 3.6 employees per patient. In spite of the increase in personnel and higher wages and salaries, payroll as a percentage of total expenses declined steadily after 1970, and by 1980 was less than one-half of total costs.

Table 5-1
U.S. Nonfederal Short-Term Hospitals—Selected Data, 1950–1983

	1950	1960	1970	1975	1980	1983	Percentage Increase 1950–1983	Percentage Increase 1970–1983
Total civilian resident population (millions)	150.80	178.20	205.10	216.00	217.70	233.70	55.0	13.9
Number of hospitals	5,031	5,407	5,859	5,979	5,904	5,783	14.9	-1.3
Number of beds (thousands)	505	639	848	947	992	1,018	101.6	20.0
Beds per 1,000 populations	3.35	3.59	4.13	4.38	4.56	4.36	30.1	-1.1
Admissions (thousands)	16,663	22,970	29,252	33,519	36,198	36,152	117.0	23.6
Admissions per 1,000 population	110.50	128.90	142.60	155.20	159.00	154.70	40.0	8.5
Average daily census (thousands)	372	477	622	708	748	749	101.3	20.4
Patient days per 1,000 population	895	980	1,169	1,195	1,199	1,176	31.4	0.1
Occupancy (%)	73.70	74.70	78.00	74.80	75.40	73.50	-0.3	-5.8
Average length of stay (days)	8.10	7.60	8.20	7.70	7.60	7.60	-6.2	-7.3
Total expenses (millions of $)	2,120	5,617	19,560	39,110	76,970	116,438	5,392.4	495.3
Total expenses per patient day	15.62	32.23	81.58	151.51	281.92	423.67	2,612.4	419.3
Expenses per patient stay	127.26	244.53	668.96	1,166.62	2,142.59	3,219.89	2,430.2	381.3
Expenses per patient stay (1983 $)	528.33	824.99	1,720.32	2,165.45	2,597.46	3,219.89	509.4	87.2
Expense per person	14.06	31.52	95.37	181.06	338.03	498.23	3,443.6	422.4
Expense per person (1983 $)	58.51	106.34	245.26	336.07	409.79	498.23	751.5	103.1
Full-time personnel (thousands)[a]	662	1,080	1,929	2,399	2,879	3,096	367.7	60.5
Full-time personnel per 100 patients[a]	178	226	310	339	385	413	132.0	33.2
Payroll expenses (millions of $)	1,203	3,400	11,421	20,749	37,460	55,525	4,515.5	386.2
Payroll expenses per patient day	8.86	20.08	47.63	79.00	167.00	202.03	2,180.2	324.2
Payroll expenses per patient day (1983 $)	36.79	67.72	122.49	146.63	167.00	202.03	449.1	64.9
Average payroll expense per employee	1,817	3,229	5,921	8,649	13,011	17,934	887.0	213.5
Payroll expense as percentage of total expense	56.75	60.53	58.38	53.05	48.70	47.69	-16.0	-18.3

Source: *Hospital Statistics, 1984* (Chicago: American Hospital Association, 1984), pp. xvii–xxiii.
[a]Includes part-time equivalents except in 1950.

Total expense per patient day, the hospital's average per diem cost, rose rapidly from 1950 to 1983, up a total of 2,612 percent to a level of $423.67. The slight decline in length of stay was more than offset by cost increases, and the average expense per patient stay rose 2,430 percent to $3,219.89.

An important indicator of changing hospital operations, one not shown in table 5–1, is the rising number of institutions with specialized technical facilities. Virtually all nonfederal, short-term hospitals have a clinical laboratory and diagnostic x-ray equipment compared with 76 and 86 percent respectively in 1946. The percentage of hospitals with registered pharmacists increased from 63 percent in 1967 to 96 percent in 1983.[3] Moreover, many services are now available that were unknown a generation ago. Thus, in 1983, 70.8 percent of hospitals have ultrasound equipment, 15.8 percent perform cardiac catheterizations, and 78.9 percent have ambulatory surgery facilities.

Types of Hospitals

There are a number of different kinds of hospitals. This chapter does not consider long-term hospitals, nor does it discuss federal hospitals because they are not generally accessible to the general public. Even within the designation "nonfederal, short-term," there are several classifications. The following table shows the 1983 distribution according to ownership and relative size.[4]

| | Percentage | | |
Type of Hospital	Hospitals	Beds	Full-time Personnel
Voluntary	57.6	70.3	73.2
Proprietary	13.0	9.2	6.9
State and local government	29.5	20.5	19.9
Total	100.0	100.0	100.0

The state and local hospitals are owned and operated by municipalities, counties, or states. In heavily populated or urbanized areas, they tend to serve mainly the indigent and low-income patients. Charges have been traditionally related to income. However, in some localities, the county hospital is the only hospital within a broad geographic area and so serves the entire population.

The proprietary hospital is a business enterprise, usually owned and operated by groups of doctors in connection with their medical practice, but sometimes as a separate business activity. Such hospitals may by owned by other private investors.[5] Increasingly, corporations are operating nationwide chains of proprietary hospitals, raising the likelihood of increasing seller concentration in this element of the hospital industry.

The proprietary hospitals are guided primarily by profit considerations in determining the range of services offered and the prices to be charged for these services. Thus, they exhibit behavior similar to private firms in other industries and attempt to maximize profits. Generally these hospitals limit their services to full-pay patients and avoid the medically indigent.

Some of the nonprofit aspects of the voluntary hospital are disappearing. The charity patient is more likely to go elsewhere, and, because of Medicaid and Medicare, there are fewer charity patients. Increasingly, the voluntary hospital expects to be reimbursed at least at the level of costs for services rendered. Both proprietary and voluntary hospitals hope to produce a profit in the sense that current operating revenues will exceed costs. The difference between them lies in what is done with the surplus. None of the voluntary hospitals' surplus may be distributed to the owners; it is all ultimately reinvested in expansion, renovation, or improvement.

Hospital Expenditures

In the recent past, hospital expenditures have grown rapidly. From 1968 to 1983, community hospital expenditures increased at an average annual rate of 14.7 percent. This growth has been more rapid than that of consumer prices for the economy as a whole, which increased at an average annual rate of approximately 8 percent during these years, while total personal consumption expenditures rose at an annual rate of 11 percent.

Federal outlays for hospital care under the Medicare and Medicaid programs, which together presently account for about 40 percent of community hospital revenues, have increased even more rapidly. From 1968 to 1983 their annual rate of increase averaged 17 percent.

In the absence of effective hospital cost containment, hospital expenditures were projected by the Congressional Budget Office to nearly double between fiscal year 1979 and fiscal year 1984. Annual expenditures were expected to rise by about $63 billion (from $66 billion to $129 billion), while federal Medicare and Medicaid outlays for hospital care were expected to increase by about $31 billion (from $23 billion to $54 billion). Based on preliminary data, these projections were accurate.[6]

As expenditures rise, taxes or deficits must increase to meet the correspondingly higher outlays from federal health programs. While business and individuals must pay higher premiums for health insurance plans, fewer resources are available for other types of private and public consumption. However, reallocation of resources from one sector to another is typical in a dynamic economy. More resources are allocated to the computer industry each year, for example. Why then is there a concern about additional resources flowing into the hospital sector?

The concern stems from doubts about whether the increases in expenditures have resulted in concomitant gains in the value of medical services. Many experts claim that too many resources are being allocated to health services in general and hospital care in particular. They assert that there is waste (partially caused by duplication of facilities and poor management) and that some services have little or no effectiveness and, thus, are unnecessary. Technical ignorance on the part of patients, and the fact that much medical expense is borne by third parties such as governments and insurance companies, cause competition to be weaker in the health sector than in other markets. Since the patient frequently does not pay directly for services rendered, the normal market test—whether a service can be sold at a given price—is not applicable.

Components of Hospital Expenditure Increases

Hospital expenditure increases are made up of four basic components.

1. The higher prices hospitals pay for the goods and services used in the delivery of care. These hospital inputs include food, fuel, supplies, labor, and capital goods.
2. The increased use of hospital services. The number of hospital admissions and days of hospital care have been rising. Outpatient visits also increased rapidly until 1983.
3. The changing character—often referred to as the "service intensity"—of hospital services. Hospitals continually add services and more frequently deliver existing ones such as lab tests and x-rays.
4. Slow productivity increases. Private firms rely on productivity gains to keep increases in product prices below gains in wages. If hospital productivity advances relative to wage increases are smaller than in other industries, prices of hospital services and expenditures on hospital care will increase more rapidly than expenditures in other sectors.[7]

Although increases in the prices of hospital inputs account for over half of the growth in hospital expenditures, increases in utilization and intensity rather than staff salaries have been responsible for the remaining rapid increase in total outlays for hospital services.

Hospital utilization increased faster than the amount that could be explained by the growth and aging of the population. As indicated by adjusted admissions (a measure combining admissions and outpatient visits), utilization increased at an average annual rate of 2.8 percent. Meanwhile, population (adjusted for the higher utilization associated with the aging of the population) grew by only 1.3 percent a year. Net intensity increased at an average annual rate of 3.2 percent from 1969 to 1979.[8]

As for payroll costs, a recent study compared gains in hospital employees' real wages to wage gains of workers of similar quality in other sectors. It found that during the 1960s, hospital workers' real wages rose faster than those of comparable employee groups. However, during the 1970s, hospital workers' wages failed to keep pace with earnings of workers at similar skill levels and in fact even failed to keep pace with inflation.[9]

Causes of Rapid Expenditure Increases

Four major reasons have been suggested to explain why hospital expenditures have been growing more rapidly than can be accounted for by the increased prices of hospital inputs and by population increases. These reasons include a lack of competition in the market for hospital services, new technological developments, rising real incomes, and the changing health status of the population.[10] Changing consumer tastes and preferences, while difficult to precisely specify, also affect the growth in hospital expenditures.

Lack of Competition. The hospital industry is much less competitive than other industries. Since over 90 percent of hospital bills are paid for by third parties such as Medicare, Medicaid, and private insurance companies, patients usually have little immediate financial interest in the cost of their care. Further, few patients or doctors have much information as to whether particular services delivered by a hospital are worth their cost, a situation probably made worse by the extensiveness of third-party payment.

Health insurance raises the demand for hospital care in two ways. From the perspective of the patient, the net price of hospital care is reduced so that financial deterrence declines. Thus, for a given illness, patients are less reluctant to either go to or remain in a hospital. They are more likely to insist that their physicians employ all the diagnostic or therapeutic procedures available. With the physician acting on behalf of the patient, insurance gives strong inducements to order additional services. It removes a deterrent to ignoring costs in ordering services that might benefit the patient. Moreover, under the fee-for-service system of financing, insurance increases the income physicians may obtain from performing services. Since the balancing of costs and benefits of additional services is less likely to occur, insurance results in higher and more rapidly rising expenditures on hospital care than would occur in its absence.

Increased demand for medical care associated with greater insurance coverage can cause increases in service intensity. As the net price to the patient declines, individuals demand higher quality care and more amenities such as better food, more nurses, and superior accommodations. The increasing insurance coverage, by reducing the price elasticity of demand, allows the provider to charge higher prices without reducing total utilization.

The new revenues may then be used to obtain new equipment, hire more staff, and improve patient amenities.

Present tax laws worsen the situation by the way in which health insurance is treated. The exclusion from taxable income of all employer contributions to employee health plans gives employees a strong incentive to sacrifice money wages for more extensive insurance coverage than they would purchase with after-tax dollars. The additional insurance further reduces incentives to economize in the use of medical services. Furthermore, where employers offer a choice of health plans, as for example, between traditional insurance and enrollment in a less expensive HMO, employees usually do not benefit financially from choosing the low-cost plan, thus reducing incentives to choose such plans.

Although hospitals traditionally have shown little concern about the prices charged patients, they are concerned about attracting physicians who are the source of patient admissions. Since physicians prefer to practice at hospitals that offer a full range of modern services, hospitals often duplicate each others' facilities. This often results in excess capacity and inefficiency.

Technological Developments. The adoption of new technologies has also contributed to rising expenditures on hospital care. One fairly recent innovation, the coronary bypass operation, costs $10,000 or more. Another, electronic fetal monitoring, is now performed in roughly half of obstetrical cases at a total cost of over $400 million per year. While new technology usually benefits patients and increases hospital productivity, it is often embodied in new services that are additions to, rather than replacements for, existing services. Consequently, new technology often increases the utilization of hospital care, an important factor in the growth of expenditures by hospitals.

However, not all technological advances raise costs. For example, a new drug treatment, Indocin I.V., that became available in February 1985 could save thousands of premature babies from undergoing heart surgery and could cut hospital bills by a minimum of $4,000 per infant. The U.S. Food and Drug Administration has approved this intravenous form of a widely used antiarthritic drug, for treatment of the condition known as patent ductus arteriosus, or PDA, a malfunction that can cause the newborn infant severe heart failure. This drug treatment will eliminate the necessity for surgery in at least two-thirds of the cases in which surgery has traditionally been performed. About 16,500 babies have been operated on for PDA in recent years.[11]

An important issue is the relationship between the introduction of cost-increasing technology and third-party payment. It is maintained that third-party payment has increased the rate of adoption of such technology. If this is correct, then much of the increase in hospital expenditures associated with new technology is another manifestation of the third-party financing system. However, an alternative position is that technological advances are exogenous, or not influenced by insurance. Indeed, the possibility exists that expensive third-party financing is a response to technological developments that have made hospital care more costly.

Rising Personal Income. As people's real incomes grow, they tend to purchase more goods and services of all kinds. Some, especially the uninsured, may demand more hospital care as their incomes rise. Others may purchase more health insurance, leading in turn to increased expenditures for hospital care. However, with over 90 percent of hospital bills already covered by insurance, rising incomes have little additional potential to increase hospital expenditures.

Changing Health Status. Trends in the population's health status also influence expenditures through changes in the utilization and intensity of hospital care. The aging of the population should increase both utilization and intensity. Changing lifestyles may also affect health status and hospital expenditures. However, increasing education and better nonhospital medical care may improve health and reduce inpatient hospital use.

Hospital Cost Containment

The growth of expenditures on medical care, and particularly hospital care, has led several recent administrations to propose limits on hospital outlays or other restrictions on medical spending increases. President Richard Nixon launched his economic stabilization program on August 15, 1971, by freezing all prices and wages for ninety days. His Phase II controls, which lasted from November 1971 to April 30, 1974, contained detailed and complex limits on the allowable increase in revenue per patient day of hospital care.[12]

The 1978 budget of Gerald Ford requested Congress to limit the rate of increase in per diem reimbursements to hospitals and physicians participating in both the Medicare and Medicaid programs.[13] The limit was to be 7 percent or the actual rate of increase in the previous year, whichever was smaller. However, President Carter withdrew the Ford proposals because he felt they would create a lower standard of care for the poor, the aged, and the disabled than for other patients, resulting in a two-class, discriminatory health care system.

As an alternative to the Ford budget initiatives, the Carter administration proposed a limit on the increase in total inpatient revenues of nonfederal, short-term hospitals. This limit would apply to all patients and not only to those covered by Medicare and Medicaid.[14] On November 15, 1979, the House of Representatives rejected the Carter bill and voted instead to establish a national commission to study the problem of hospital costs.

Upon entering office in 1981, the Reagan administration declared that it would undertake various measures to control the increase in expenditures

Table 5–2
Characteristics of Eight State Regulatory Programs

State	Regulatory Agency	General Methodology	Funding Source	Frequency of Review
Connecticut	Independent commission	Budget review, formula	State; federal grants	Annually and at time of change
Maryland	Independent commission	Budget review, negotiation, formula	State; federal grants	Annually and at time of change
Massachusetts	Independent commission	Budget review, formula	State; federal grants	At time of change
New Jersey	State department of health	Budget review, negotiation	State; federal grants	Annually
New York	State executive branch offices	Formula	State	Annually and at change
Rhode Island	State government, hospital association, Blue Cross	Budget review, negotiation	Not available	Annually
Washington	Independent commission	Budget review	State; hospitals' federal grants	Annually
Wisconsin	State hospital rate program	Budget review	Blue Cross; Medicaid program	At time of change

Source: Unpublished data from the American Hospital Association.

under the Medicaid and Medicare programs. Besides desiring cuts in benefits, Reagan officials expressed support for measures designed to increase competition in the delivery of care partly by making patients and health care providers more cost-conscious.

At the same time, Congress tried to slow the rate of increase in medical expenditures by issuing regulations that required states to attempt to prevent duplication of medical facilities. By 1980, all states except Louisiana required health care providers to obtain a certificate-of-need (CON) from the local health systems agency before making a capital expenditure greater than $100,000 to $150,000. If the provider made such an expenditure without a CON, the institution was prohibited from receiving reimbursement from Medicaid or Medicare. In principle, a CON is granted only if there are no facilities in the area offering similar services, or if existing facilities are operating at or above utilization levels established by federal and state guidelines.

Evaluation studies show that CON programs slow the increase in the number of beds, but that the funds saved are simply allocated to new services and equipment so that there is no demonstrable effect on overall hospital costs. Moreover, savings in CON programs that were begun some time ago (so that the accumulation of experience might lead to improved results) are no greater than in new programs. In addition, the prevention of all duplication would achieve only modest, one-time savings, and would not affect subsequent rates of increase in costs.[15] Given these findings, and because of an antiregulation bias, in 1982 the Reagan administration sought to terminate the CON programs, but Congress extended the authorization through 1983.

Meanwhile, state governments have been experimenting with cost-containment methods. By 1980, eight states had introduced mandatory programs to reduce the rate of growth of hospital expenditures.[16] These programs control hospital charges, third-party payment rates, and/or total hospital revenue, and hospitals are forced to absorb any costs beyond their allowed reimbursement levels.

The state programs differ considerably in terms of organizational structure, methods of controlling reimbursement rates, types of payers covered, resources devoted to regulatory efforts, and the extent of interaction with providers and insurers. Table 5–2 lists some of the characteristics of the eight mandatory programs. Most of these programs have continued to evolve. Since this form of regulation is relatively new, there are limited administrative models to follow, and useful cost-accounting and information-collection systems did not previously exist.

Hospital Regulation in New York State—A Case Study

New York was the first state to adopt a mandatory reimbursement regulation program. There is general perception that its regulatory program places the greatest financial constraints on hospitals.

Reimbursement rates for Medicaid and Blue Cross patients (accounting for about 50 percent of total hospital revenues) are based on a complicated set of formulas and trend factors. Hospitals are divided into comparable groups based on the number of beds, services offered, and whether or not they are teaching facilities. Hospitals whose costs are above 125 percent or below 75 percent of the group mean are excluded, and a new group mean is calculated.[17] Any hospital costs above the new group mean are excluded from reimbursement unless the hospital is able to successfully appeal such a decision. The New York system also penalizes hospitals that do not achieve target occupancy rates. For example, urban hospitals are expected to achieve medical-surgical occupancy rates of 85 percent, pediatric occupancy rates of 70 percent, and maternity unit occupancy rates of 60 percent. Hospitals that have lower occupancy rates have their actual patient days adjusted to the level that would have yielded the required occupancy rate. This leads to a reduction in the per diem rate allowed since the allowed per diem rate is (roughly) obtained by dividing allowable costs by actual inpatient days plus penalty inpatient days.

The formulas are used to define base-level costs for each hospital, and trend factors reflecting inflation are used to adjust base costs to prospective reimbursement rates. These trend factors underestimate the rate of change in input prices so retroactive payments have been made. Furthermore, base-level costs have been adjusted upward very slowly.

This approach has placed severe financial pressure on hospitals throughout the state. As a whole, New York community hospitals have sustained deficits during 1976, 1977, and 1978, and about 80 percent of all New York hospitals had deficits in 1977 or 1978. The financial pressure has forced a number of hospitals into bankruptcy and has also led to hospital mergers. However, if the policy is to use financial constraints to reduce a perceived excess capacity and to limit expansion, this result is to be expected, especially in the short run.[18]

Cost Containment in States with Various Types of Regulatory Programs

Table 5–3 presents data on recent expenditures among the states classified by type of regulation. It is clear that, as a group, from 1975 to 1979 the states with mandatory regulation of hospital budgets or charges experienced a significantly lower rate of growth in total expenditures and expenditures per patient day than did the rest of the states. However, this group of states also had a significantly lower growth rate in expenditures during the 1973–1975 period, even though at that time several of these states had not yet established comprehensive reimbursement regulation procedures. During both time periods, every state in the group experienced lower expenditure growth than the mean

Table 5–3
Comparisons between Regulated and Unregulated States

States	Change in Total Expenses (%)		Change in Cost per Day (%)		Cost per Admission ($)		Personnel per Bed	
	1975–1979	1973–1975	1975–1979	1973–1975	1975	1979	1975	1979
A. States with mandatory rate regulatory programs								
Connecticut	57.4	28.6	49.8	24.9	1,233	1,835	3.00	3.32
Maryland	68.9	33.4	51.5	27.3	1,277	1,946	3.02	3.22
Massachusetts	51.7	34.3	48.9	30.6	1,495	2,286	3.31	3.55
New Jersey	57.0	38.3	52.5	27.2	1,100	1,668	2.44	2.66
New York	37.0	33.7	39.8	28.1	1,628	2,230	3.02	3.17
Rhode Island	51.0	35.5	48.1	35.5	1,288	1,916	3.41	3.77
Washington	70.0	35.0	59.4	29.8	844	1,360	2.56	2.94
Wisconsin	69.5	31.8	69.0	27.4	939	1,573	2.20	2.54
Simple means for eight-state group	57.8	33.8	52.4	28.9	1,226	1,852	2.87	3.15
B. Simple means for remaining states	80.6	38.3	70.0	31.5	867	1,464	2.39	2.65
C. Simple means for states with CON programs prior to 1975	73.9	37.3	64.0	30.9	1,003	1,611	2.54	2.81
D. Same as C excluding states in A	80.5	38.5	69.2	31.6	906	1,509	2.39	2.66
E. Means for states without CON prior to 1975	80.3	37.9	70.0	31.3	840	1,434	2.38	2.64

Source: Adapted from Paul Joskow, *Controlling Hospital Costs: The Role of Government Regulation* (Cambridge, Mass.: MIT Press, 1981), p. 146.

for the rest of the states in the population. But, on the average, the differences are much greater from 1975 to 1979 than from 1973 to 1975.

States with rate regulation programs were generally high-cost states at the time the regulatory activities became effective. Seven of the eight states with regulatory programs had higher cost per stay than the rest of the population in both 1975 and 1979. Although the difference in cost per stay between the regulated and the unregulated states has declined, the regulated states continue to exhibit on average higher cost per admission.

Such state controls appear to constrain the rate of growth of hospital costs by about 3 percent a year, but only after the programs have been in operation for at least three years.[19] These results differ greatly from the relative ineffectiveness of CON programs. One major question concerns the ability of states to sustain reimbursement limits for a considerable period of time. Will the states that have adopted controls be willing to maintain them as the difference between actual expenditures and unregulated expenditures grows? Does the political will to curb growth of hospital expenditures exist outside the states that have established controls?

Such questions are not merely academic. In 1982, for example, Massachusetts enacted legislation limiting expenditures of all hospitals to 7.5 percent below the rate of inflation.[20] This will put considerable pressure on those hospitals to increase efficiency in order to survive.

Declining Hospital Occupancy Rates and Increased Competition

A twenty-year expansion period for hospitals appears to have ended as hospitals increasingly report declining occupancy rates. Decreasing occupancy rates and reduced length of stay strongly suggest that some hospitals are coming under increased financial pressure. In today's cost-containment environment, hospital administrators are attempting to diversify and provide new revenue-generating services.

For consumers, this means shorter stays in the hospital and more outpatient services relative to inpatient services. This is even true in the case of surgical procedures that traditionally were performed on an inpatient basis. For private firms, the declining occupancy rates may mean that employee health insurance costs will rise more slowly.[21] Table 5–4 indicates the sharp drop in occupancy rates nationally and in the Washington metropolitan area.

The single most important factor in the marked change in hospital use is Medicare's new prospective payment program which is based on diagnostic-related groups. Under this DRG system, hospitals are reimbursed a fixed amount for specific medical treatments. (See chapter 4.) Basically, the DRG

Table 5–4
Hospital Bed Occupancy, 1980–1984
(First Quarter of Year, in Percent)

	1980	1981	1982	1983	1984
Nationwide	79.1	79.5	77.9	77.4	71.9
Washington metro area	83.9	84.6	83.3	84.0	77.1
Montgomery Country, Maryland	86.2	82.5	78.2	85.5	79.1
Southern Maryland	84.2	89.3	87.3	88.6	83.6
District of Columbia	84.2	84.5	84.0	83.9	76.1
Northern Virginia	81.9	83.4	82.8	80.6	73.9

Source: Calculated from Arthur Brisbane, "Hospital Occupancy Dip Sparks Income Struggle," *The Washington Post*, July 30, 1984, p. A-8.

reimbursement system provides an incentive to get a patient out of the hospital as fast as medically permissible because the reimbursement amount remains the same regardless of length of stay.

Other sources of competition among providers have also reduced occupancy levels at hospitals. These include HMOs, which emphasize preventive medicine, as well as preferred provider insurance plans in which hospitals offering relatively inexpensive services are used.

Hospitals have responded with a variety of innovations aimed at dealing with the increasingly competitive environment. Some, like the Washington Hospital Center and the National Hospital for Orthopedics and Rehabilitation in Arlington, Virginia, have diversified and formed corporate umbrellas for ventures into other fields. National Hospital has developed an HMO as well as a satellite sports medicine clinic. Washington Hospital Center has entered real estate development and established an ambulatory surgery center. It has also reduced services in other areas, laying off staff and, in 1984, closing at least 100 beds.[22]

Many hospitals are providing specialized services tailored to particular markets. For example, Suburban Hospital in Bethesda, Maryland, is offering deluxe two-room suites to its affluent patients.

The prospective payment system, which only affects the care of patients 65 years old or over, is having a broader impact. Hospitals are reducing the length of stay of those covered by private insurance. Many thought that hospitals would make up whatever money they might lose from Medicare by increasing the cost to privately insured patients, but this is not happening.

Moreover, some insurance plans and self-insured corporations are adopting cost-containment procedures. For example, the Kansas Blue Cross/Blue Shield plan, the largest insurer in the state, has told medical providers it expects the premiums it charges businesses to be unchanged in 1984, compared with average annual increases of 12 to 14 percent since 1968.[23] Under one aspect of the new policy, the Kansas plan won't pay patients, their doctors, or hospitals for inpatient care for some sixty elective surgical procedures unless a specific medical reason is given. For example, to receive reimbursement for a tonsillectomy or removal of a malignant breast tumor, a doctor must perform the procedure in a hospital's outpatient clinic or in a doctor's office. Moreover, the Kansas Blue Cross/Blue Shield plan will pay doctors an extra $50 to $100 for keeping the patient out of the hospital. Similarly, an innovative Blue Cross/Blue Shield plan now operating in a dozen states offers new mothers cash incentives of $50 to $200 and other benefits, including up to nine hours of free maid service, to leave the hospital within twenty-four hours after delivery. About one thousand to one thousand five hundred women have taken advantage of the program as of March 1985.[24]

Some doctors say the new pressure to reduce hospital utilization encourages them to reconsider how they provide care. They indicate that new technology and new programs are helping to reduce the length of some hospital stays. Thus, removal of a brain tumor five years ago typically meant a six-week hospital stay. Following surgery, the patient can now be discharged in a few days and cared for at home for the next few weeks at 10 percent of the daily cost of hospital care.

In Cleveland, Blue Cross limits the number of hospital days it pays for, providing an incentive for patients at St. Luke's to shorten hospital stays. Philadelphia area hospitals indicate new competition from nonhospital emergency and ambulatory surgery clinics. Such free-standing clinics proliferate as employers are altering insurance benefits to encourage out-of-hospital care. In Dallas, Presbyterian Hospital says inpatient admissions are down but surgery performed on an outpatient basis is up 15 to 20 percent.[25]

The DRG system greatly reduces the incentive to keep patients longer and perform extra tests. Yet, if patients are discharged faster, the result is lower occupancy rates which causes reduced revenues. The way to avoid lower occupancy is to obtain more patients.

Many hospitals around the nation are opening outpatient walk-in clinics sometimes called "doc's-in-the-box." If a patient needs hospitalization, the sponsoring hospital obtains the patient. For example, Northwestern Memorial Hospital in Chicago, a major teaching hospital, has opened a walk-in clinic at a nearby business center, plus an outpatient geriatric screening center. Any of the patients needing hospitalization are admitted directly to Northwestern. Northwestern also has agreements with two prepaid HMOs which refer patients needing hospitalization to Northwestern. The two HMOs obtain reduced charges at the hospital for their members.[26]

Some hospitals, such as St. Louis University Medical Center, have revived the house call. They hire or contract with doctors to answer house-call requests. People receiving services this way can be referred directly to the Medical Center.

In addition, many hospitals, in order to maximize revenues and keep their occupany rates high, are attempting to link up with physicians who have high admission rates by virtue of their specialty or size of practice. Hospitals retain their physicians and try to obtain others by offering better office space, low office rent in a hospital-owned medical building, or hospital equipment that the doctor wants.

Hospital Dumping

There is evidence that the financial squeeze on private hospitals resulting from Medicaid and Medicare cutbacks, as well as from declining occupancy rates which are partly the result of increased competition, is resulting in a phenomenon known as "dumping." Dumping is defined as a practice in which hospitals avoid admitting or keeping poor or uninsured patients by sending them to hospitals willing to absorb the costs.

Moreover, dumping appears to be increasing in frequency. An analysis of medical records of 103 patients transferred from private hospitals to tax-supported Highland General Hospital in Oakland, California, found that in nearly one-third of these cases the transfer placed the patient in medical jeopardy.[27] The study concluded that the transfers were made for economic rather than medical reasons because Highland's care wasn't necessarily better than that of any of the private hospitals involved. Similarly, in Dallas, indigent patients in 1984 were transferred from private hospitals to tax-supported Parkland Memorial Hospital at the rate of 200 a month, nearly three times the 1983 rate. In 1984, Cook County Hospital in Chicago admitted 6,000 emergency patients transferred from private hospitals. That was five times as many transfers as occurred in 1980.

Some states are acting to limit dumping abuses. In 1984, Florida began taxing private hospitals at a rate of 1 percent of their revenues to fund a pool to pay bills of uninsured, low-income patients. Kentucky business and health leaders formed a foundation to persuade doctors and hospitals to volunteer free care for poor patients not covered by health care plans. A telephone hotline service, begun in January 1985, arranged free care for almost twelve thousand Kentucky patients in its first six weeks.[28]

Hospital Advertising

As occupancy rates decline, hospitals are turning to advertising as a means of obtaining patients. Although this phenomenon is too recent to evaluate its success, one should remember that generally a patient is referred to a hospital by his personal physician, who may or may not have hospital privileges at a particular hospital. The purchase of hospital services is not the same thing as buying an automobile. You cannot just shop around.

A Case Study of Maryland

To fill underused facilities, Maryland hospitals are engaging in extensive advertising. The advertisements often describe those hospital programs that may produce the most revenue and result in more efficient use of facilities, such as maternity services, drug-alcohol-tobacco addiction treatment, and preventive medicine/fitness activities.

Carroll County General Hospital sends out $2-off coupons for its weekend emergency room clinic in a mass-mailing advertising pack. Memorial Hospital in Easton advertised that its patients could get refunds for substandard services such as cold meals and slow reception, but not for below average medical results. Franklin Square Hospital publicized its programs in regional editions of *Time* and *Sports Illustrated*. St. Joseph's saturated the community with full-color brochures and a newsletter promoting its facilities, while Children's Hospital printed a newspaper supplement to show that its activities are not limited to pediatric services. Mercy Hospital in Baltimore spent $65,000 on a billboard, radio, and television campaign to attract females working downtown to its Women Care programs. Mount Sinai pointed out that it has converted a former athletic club into a health and fitness center. Free-standing emergency centers are also advertising, with some offering an introductory discount for walk-in patients who would otherwise go to a hospital clinic.[29]

There is an economic basis for the increased advertising. Maryland hospital administrators are aware that there will soon be an estimated surplus of 5,000 hospital beds—20 percent of the state's total—and that hospitals with the highest occupancy rates will be in the strongest economic position.

Major insurers such as Blue Cross are attempting to use only hospitals that have achieved successful cost-containment policies. The State Health Resources Planning Commission is preparing a plan for cutbacks at specific hospitals. When the Planning Commission reaches a decision regarding what to do with the surplus beds, "You are going to see a lot more advertising," predicts Gary Michael, director of public relations at Mercy Hospital. "Desperate people do desperate things."[30]

Marketing Issues

Physicians still determine where patients will be hospitalized in most cases. Price advertising by hospitals does not seem practical because insurance companies and purchasers of group health insurance will make cost comparisons themselves.

For which services are hospitals likely to compete with each other? Drug- and alcohol-addiction programs are expanding in terms of both inpatient and outpatient care. "Wellness" services, aimed at business clients, are growing.

Some hospitals are now publicizing new programs that meet previously unrecognized health problems such as sleeping disorders or podiatry issues for the elderly.

Most hospitals have a maternity ward, but that department often loses money because the volume is too low for revenues to equal the cost of the facilities. Attracting more women through marketing and advertising may make the unit more profitable. Marketing costs can be relatively small. A 2 percent increase in maternity cases, or 32 new babies per year, would pay for the entire advertising program for Women Care at Mercy Hospital. In the first two weeks of an advertising campaign the hospital got 50 inquiries from women seeking referral to a physician (from the panel of doctors with privileges at Mercy), an indication of advertising success.

Because obstetricians have privileges at several hospitals, the woman can typically choose the hospital in which she wants to deliver. If she is satisfied with the services, she may continue to utilize the institution. In order to obtain maternity patients, hospitals have developed birthing centers that look like the home bedroom and may even feature champagne and gourmet dinners for the new parents, natural birth options, and brass cradles for the newborn.[31] (See chapter 8.) Selling hospital care should not be like selling travel on a luxury liner, but the differences may be shrinking.

The For-Profit Hospital

The exact dimensions of the for-profit sector of providers of health services are unknown. Rough estimates have put the gross revenues of the investor-owned health care industry as high as $40 billion.[32]

In 1984, 1,215 hospitals in the United States—about 20 percent of community hospitals—were owned or operated by chains. Between 1978 and 1984, the number of hospitals owned by for-profit hospital chains (that is, those owning at least three hospitals) more than doubled, going from 438 to 890 hospitals.[33] However, during this period, the total number of hospitals decreased slightly and the number of independently owned for-profit hospitals declined rapidly due to many being purchased by chains.[34]

Most of the firms that own chains of hospitals (as well as those that own other kinds of health service facilities) were established since 1970. They have grown by means of the purchase, construction, and contract management of institutions, and by buying smaller chains. The increasing size of these companies has itself attracted attention. Multihospital systems or chains enable some hospitals to specialize in cancer therapy and others in open-heart surgery. Because transportation costs are minimal, the unoccupied beds in one hospital may be filled by overflow patients from nearby hospitals belonging to that chain.

Multihospital systems or hospital chains are competitive and in some cases appear to allocate scarce resources more efficiently and contain costs comparatively effectively in those areas where government regulation and imposed reimbursement controls have been ineffective. Among the successful chains of smaller urban and rural nonprofit hospitals is the Intermountain Health Care, Inc. (IHC) system based in Salt Lake City, Utah. It has thirty hospital affiliates in twenty-seven cities and towns in Utah, Nevada, Colorado, and Wyoming. IHC patients pay 28 percent less per admission than the national average and 18 percent less than the regional average, while remaining hospitalized an average of 5.1 days, or 2.3 days less than the national average. IHC's $30 million in bonds carry a AA + rating from *Standard and Poor's*. This means that the chain saves $1.6 million annually in interest charges over a company with an AA rating, and $3.8 million over one with an A rating.[35] Additionally, IHC carries its own malpractice insurance and workers' compensation for up to the first $100,000 per occurrence and, through Mutual Insurance Ltd., obtains further coverage under an umbrella policy.

The Associated Hospital System was recently formed as a network of hospital chains, and has given its members even greater power in negotiating volume buying. AH contracts average 10 percent to 15 percent better savings than contracts negotiated by individual member systems.[36]

Although growth of profit-making hospitals is discouraged by the laws of some states, the number of their beds is growing. Some claim that for-profit hospitals generally handle less complex cases requiring relatively inexpensive equipment, and tend to specialize. Thus, they are often accused of skimming off the more profitable types of hospital cases.[37]

About twenty-five multihospital systems own or manage over 50 percent of all the community hospitals in the United States. Most of these conglomerates are nonprofit. However, several hospital stocks are listed on the New York Stock Exchange and the American Stock Exchange, including the two largest, Humana and Hospital Corporation of America. In 1980, Humana had a 33.6 percent return on equity and five-year average earnings per share of 34.4 percent, while Hospital Corporation of America, the largest chain of all, had 18.0 percent and 27.6 percent respectively. These indicators of profitability were well above the comparative all-industry medians of 16.1 percent and 14.3 percent respectively.[38] Primarily well known in the hotel and motel business, Hyatt Hotels and Ramada Inns have also entered the hospital sector.

From mid-1966 until 1972, Medicare assured hospitals an income to cover costs including interest payments, depreciation allowances, and a "reasonable return on equity." The latter incentive was eliminated in 1972, but by then the proprietary chains, many with motel experience, had entered the market and they managed the hotel-type hospital services more efficiently than did the nonprofit hospitals.

Mergers and Acquisitions

Some large city hospitals in difficult financial circumstances have been taken over by for-profit management. For example, Cook County Hospital of Chicago is managed by Hyatt Medical Management Services, Inc.[39] Others are being managed by nearby university medical schools such as Tulane University and Boston University Medical Schools. Large city hospitals with many poor patients can offer medical schools what other hospitals cannot: an assured flow of patients willing to be "teaching" or "research" patients.

For-profit health companies are also buying, leasing, and merging with university hospitals. Humana is leasing the University of Louisville Hospital and plans to construct a $40 million teaching hospital on the campus of University of Chicago Medical School. American Medical International, headquartered in Beverly Hills, with 115 hospitals in the U.S., has bought St. Joseph Hospital in Omaha, the 539-bed Catholic teaching hospital of Creighton University, for $100 million. Nashville-based Hospital Corporation of America is buying 760-bed Wesley Medical Center in Wichita, a research center associated with Health Frontiers, a not-for-profit health care system serving south-central Kansas.

For university teaching hospitals, the incentive for these arrangements is the need for capital to renovate decaying facilities and purchase state of the art medical equipment. A nuclear-magnetic resource scanner, for example, today's most advanced diagnostic tool, costs $2 million.[40] Hospital corporations have better access to capital than nonprofits since federal funds for buildings and equipment have been reduced and charity is unable to provide sufficient money to take up the slack.

For hospital chains, affiliation with a university medical center is a way to enhance a reputation for high quality care. Moreover, the teaching hospital link encourages doctors in the community who have privileges at the medical center to send less severely ill patients to other hospitals in the chain.

In order to limit cost increases, some nonprofit hospitals have formed multihospital systems to save on bulk purchases of such diverse items as drugs, blood, hospital linens, and malpractice insurance. Together they also engage in the type of capital planning routinely practiced by for-profit hospitals. Large urban hospitals are also exploring the relationship between specialization and cost containment; and many consequently no longer believe that it is necessary for every hospital to have each new type of costly medical technology and to cover all medical specialties.

Some hospital chains are starting health insurance plans. Humana believes it can succeed because it controls the source of 60 percent of all medical bills, the hospital. As one Humana executive indicated, "The one feature of our product that is clearly understood by employers is that because we own and operate hospitals we can control costs."[41] However, Blue Cross/Blue

Shield questions whether Humana and other health care providers have the resources to compete with the big insurers. For instance, Blue Cross has contracted with thirty-five hospitals to provide discount care in the Los Angeles area alone. Humana has but five hospitals in all of California.

Will a for-profit chain with a limited number of hospitals in an area be able to attract the participation it needs from employers? To expand their hospital networks to adequate size, the chains must contract with facilities they don't own, leaving them with the same cost-containment problems as traditional insurers.

Possible Problems Caused by the Growth of the For-Profit Hospital Sector

Those who are concerned about the benefits of a growing for-profit sector in health care raise several issues. These include public perceptions of the medical profession, the importance and determinants of trust in the doctor-patient relationship, and arrangements between physicians and the institutions where medical care is provided.

The type of relationship between physicians and medical facilities can cause concern about the possible tainting of the physician's role as it pertains to the patient. One difficulty is physician ownership of the hospitals, nursing homes, and radiology centers to which they make referrals. The physician with an economic interest in the full utilization of a facility may face conflicting pressures when evaluating patients' needs for the type of service that the facility provides. Moreover, there are situations in which physicians enter into incentive arrangements with institutions such that the institution rewards the physician for making patient care decisions that benefit the institution. One example is the practice of leasing office space to physicians at rates that depend on the number of patients the physician admits to the hospital.

A second set of problems relates to the effects of the growth of for-profit health care corporations on other parts of the medical care system, particularly medical research, medical education, and health care for the poor. In the past, all of these activities have been subsidized by revenues from the provision of services to paying or insured patients, who were charged more than the cost of services rendered. If such care is provided by for-profit firms, some observers are concerned that these activities will be deemphasized. It should be remembered that for-profit hospital chains are accountable to their stockholders, while a nonprofit hospital and teaching center answers to its medical school and community. While successful for-profit firms pay taxes, there is no reason to assume such revenue will be used to support medical research and teaching, let alone health care for the uninsured.

Finally, there are concerns regarding whether the for-profit institutions are really more efficient than their nonprofit counterparts. Although some studies have begun to appear,[42] and more are in progress, comparisons of cost and efficiency in for-profit and not-for-profit health care institutions are difficult to interpret without better information than presently exists about costs and productivity in hospitals, and the comparability of patient populations served by different institutions.

Veterans Administration Hospitals

The Reagan administration is considering proposals to restrict veterans' health benefits and limit expenditure increases in the veterans health care program both now and in the future. One reason is that the number of veterans age 65 or over will reach a peak of 9 million in the year 2000.[43] That is three times the number who were 65 or over in 1980. The VA spent $8.5 billion on medical care in fiscal year 1984, and has received a $9.1 billion appropriation for medical care in the 1985 fiscal year. It has projected its cost to be $13.6 billion in 1990.[44]

At present, a veteran who reaches age 65 is automatically eligible for free medical care on demand, without regard to financial need, if space is available in Veterans Administration hospitals and nursing homes. Reagan administration officials are considering proposals to charge veterans at least a nominal amount for health care services and to make benefits contingent upon financial need. In addition, the administration wants to limit benefits for veterans seeking treatment for illnesses and disabilities unrelated to their military service. Other proposals under study would encourage the use of private contractors to provide support services and perhaps health care at veterans' installations; would scale back plans for new nursing homes and hospitals; and would eliminate scheduled increases in spending for the Veterans Administration's Department of Medicine and Surgery.

Most veterans aged 65 and over are eligible for Medicare. However, veterans' health benefits are more comprehensive than Medicare recipients', and they have become increasingly attractive as Medicare requires beneficiaries to pay a growing share of program costs. Further cutbacks in Medicare would probably increase the demand for veterans' health benefits.

Government Regulation and Substandard Care

The federal government has inaugurated a program intended to require doctors and hospitals to eliminate "avoidable deaths" and "substandard care." The American Hospital Association and other national medical organizations have criticized the usefulness of the program.

Under the program, the federally financed agencies that review Medicare spending in most states are presently signing contracts with the Department of Health and Human Services. The contracts require them, for example, to assure that doctors and hospitals reduce "unnecessary" heart attack deaths, postoperative complications, and amputations by specific numbers in the next two years. Officials with the Department of Health and Human Services indicate that the numerical goals are based on studies in each state which indicate how many hospital patients may have died unnecessarily or encountered complications that could have been avoided. (The studies never have been made public.) The new program applies only to Medicare patients, but its effects probably would be felt in the care of most hospital patients.

The review agencies, called Professional Review Organizations (PROs), were established by the federal government twelve years ago in order to reduce Medicare spending. Since 1972, one or more of these agencies in almost every state has employed hundreds of doctors and nurses to review the care given to hospital patients who were Medicare beneficiaries. The reviews have been undertaken to determine whether Medicare money was spent properly and to ascertain if the patients received care of appropriate quality.

The American Medical Peer Review Association, which represents the federally financed agencies and the American Hospital Association, says the new goals are based on unreliable data and will be difficult to meet. The newly signed contract for Kentucky, as an example, requires the review agency to reduce the number of deaths which occur in Kentucky hospitals "with the principal diagnosis [of heart attack] by 20 percent on or before October 31, 1985."[45] Mississippi's new contract says the agency must ensure that the state's hospitals perform thirty-five fewer "avoidable" above-the-knee and below-the-knee amputations in the next two years. West Virginia's PRO is required to reduce by 1,631 the number of unnecessary hospital readmissions resulting from substandard care provided during prior admissions according to the state's contract.

The agencies are to encourage these changes by threatening to withhold Medicare payments to doctors and hospitals. Moreover, if the contractual objectives are not met, the government can refuse to pay the state agencies, or it can renegotiate their contracts with another agency. At present, each review agency is administered by a physician. However, the law indicates that if medical groups are unwilling or unable to fulfill the objectives, insurance companies would be permitted to bid for the contracts. The possibility of doctors' performances being judged by persons who are not similarly trained is viewed unfavorably by the medical community.

Andrew Wilber, executive vice president of the American Medical Peer Review Association, says the federal goals are unrealistic. He indicates the great difficulty in reviewing death certificates and determining which particular deaths were unnecessary. Jack Owen, executive vice president of the American Hospital Association, says, "The delivery of medical care has never lent itself to arbitrary and rigid numerical quotas." He calls the goals intrusive and unrealistic and indicates that they will be extremely difficult to achieve.[46]

The public is now able to compare hospitals for their safety and effectiveness under a new law that opens to scrutiny previously undisclosed government evaluations. The new regulations, which went into effect in May 1985, stipulate that the public is entitled to examine hospital review data compiled by Medicare's Peer Review Organizations and obtain the peer review evaluations of the hospitals.[47] These PROs are, in effect, Medicare's hospital examiners. Their reports, which now are public information, are sent to the Department of Health and Human Services (DHHS), which oversees Medicare.

Some hospitals have argued that the statistics could be misleading. Mortality figures, for example, may show higher death rates for a particular hospital because it treats large numbers of elderly patients, not because of a lower quality of care. But DHHS indicates hospitals will be protected by a provision in the law that they be given advance notice of information being released. The hospitals can then write their own explanation, which would be released with the data.

Summary

Hospital statistics indicate the average patient's hospital bill was nearly $3,220 in 1983, as compared to $127 in 1950. In no other segment of the health care industry have costs risen so rapidly.

The most important single factor accounting for increases in hospital expenditures is rises in the prices of hospital inputs. Increases in utilization and intensity of services rendered are of less importance.

Because of rapid expenditure increases, both state and federal governments have developed a number of cost-containment approaches. Among the states, New York has the most comprehensive regulatory program, but there is evidence that it is too strict, as most New York hospitals lost money soon after its implementation.

Most hospitals have experienced declining occupancy rates in the last several years, partly due to competition from walk-in clinics and health maintenance organizations. One response to reduced utilization of hospitals has been increased advertising. However, since personal physicians admit patients only to those hospitals in which they have admitting privileges, the effects of advertising are unclear.

The for-profit hospital sector is growing rapidly, particularly in the case of corporate hospital chains, which not only own hospitals, but also manage nonprofit hospitals. The rate of growth of this phenomena appears to be accelerating as for-profit chains lease or purchase academic teaching hospitals.

There is concern that for-profit hospitals may pay less attention to medical research and education than nonprofit hospitals do. In addition, for-profit hospitals may exhibit less concern for poor patients than voluntary hospitals will.

The Reagan administration is considering ways to restrict veterans' health benefits, particularly those of older veterans. Because benefits for veterans over age 65 are more comprehensive than Medicare, further reductions in Medicare benefits will tend to increase demand for veterans' health services.

The federal government has established numerical goals or quotas in regard to reducing "unnecessary" deaths among Medicare patients. Organized medicine is strongly opposed to these new regulations.

Notes

1. See Karen Davis and Louise Russell, "The Substitution of Hospital Outpatient Care for Inpatient Care," *Review of Economics and Statistics* 54, no. 2 (May 1972):109–20, for an interesting econometric study of this issue.

2. *Hospitals Statistics, 1984 Edition* (Chicago: American Hospital Association, 1984), p. xvii.

3. Ibid., p. 193.

4. Ibid., p. 6.

5. Herman Somers and Ann Somers, *Medicare and the Hospitals: Issues and Prospects* (Washington, D.C.: The Brookings Institution, 1967), p. 49.

6. Congressional Budget Office, *Controlling Rising Hospital Costs* (Washington, D.C.: U.S. Government Printing Office, 1979), p. ix.

7. Ibid., p. 2.

8. Congressional Budget Office, *Controlling Rising Hospital Costs*, p. 5.

9. F.A. Sloan and B. Steinwald, "Wage Setting in the Hospital Industry—Evidence from the 60s to 70s," Final Report Grant No. HS02 590, prepared for the National Center for Health Services Research (Washington, D.C.: National Center for Health Services Research, 1979).

10. Congressional Budget Office, *Controlling Rising Hospital Costs*, p. 4.

11. Sue Miller, "Drug Avoids Infant Heart Surgery," *The Evening Sun* (Baltimore), February 19, 1985, p. A-1.

12. For details on these controls, see Paul Ginsberg, "Inflation and the Economic Stabilization Program," in Michael Zublsoff, ed.,) *Health: A Victim or a Cause of Inflation?* (New York: Prodist for the Milbank Memorial Fund, 1976), pp. 31–51.

13. *The Budget of the United States Government, Fiscal Year 1978*, p. 159 (Washington, D.C.: U.S. Government Printing Office).

14. Congressional Budget Office, *The Hospital Cost Containment Act of 1977: An Analysis of the Administration's Proposal*, prepared for the Subcommittee on Health and Scientific Research on the Senate Committee on Human Resources, 95th Cong., 10th sess. (Washington, D.C.: U.S. Government Printing Office, 1977), p. 6.

15. David Salkever and Thomas Bice, *Hospital Certificate-of-Need Controls: Impact on Investment, Costs and Use* (Washington, D.C.: American Enterprise Institute for Public Policy Research, 1979), p. 75; and William Schwartz, "The Regulation Strategy for Controlling Hospital Costs," *New England Journal of Medicine* 305, no. 21 (November 19, 1981):1249.

16. Craig Coelen and Daniel Sullivan, "An Analysis of the Effect of Prospective Reimbursement Programs on Hospital Expenditures," *Health Care Financing Review* 2, no. 2 (Winter 1981):1–40.

17. Paul Joskow, *Controlling Hospital Costs: The Role of Government Regulation* (Cambridge, Mass.: MIT Press, 1981), p. 118.

18. Joskow, op. cit., p. 119.

19. John Iglehart, "Health Policy Report: New Jersey's Experiment with DRG-based Hospital Reimbursement," *New England Journal of Medicine* 307, no. 26 (December 23, 1982):1655–60.

20. "A New System for Hospital Payment: The Massachusetts Plan," *National Journal* 14 (August 21, 1982):1488–89; and Brian Biles et al., "Hospital Cost Inflation Under State Rate-Setting Programs," *New England Journal of Medicine* 303, no. 19 (September 18, 1980):666.

21. Arthur Brisbane, "Hospital Occupancy Dip Sparks Income Struggle," *The Washington Post*, July 30, 1984, p. A-1.

22. Ibid., p. A-8.

23. Michael Waldholz, "New Views About Care in Hospitals Lead to Slower Rise in Health Costs," *Wall Street Journal*, October 14, 1984, p. 1.

24. Steven Findlay, "New Moms Get Bonus to Go Home Early," *USA Today*, March 1–3, 1985, p. A-1.

25. "Hospital Use Drops as Health Insurance Plans Try to Stem Cost Increases," *Wall Street Journal*, September 20, 1984, p. A-1.

26. Spencer Rich, "Hospitals are Competing for Patients," *The Washington Post*, October 13, 1984, p. B-1.

27. "Hospitals in Cost Squeeze 'Dump' More Patients Who Can't Pay Bills," *Wall Street Journal*, March 8, 1985, p. 33.

28. Ibid.

29. Michael Burns, "Medicine Avenue/Madison Avenue," *The Baltimore Sun*, November 17, 1984, p. A-1.

30. Ibid.

31. Ibid., p. N-3.

32. Arnold Rilman, "The New Medical-Industrial Complex," *New England Journal of Medicine* 303, no. 21 (October 23, 1980):963–70.

33. "As Controversy Mounts Over Hospitals-for-Profit," *U.S. News and World Report*, December 10, 1984, p. 61.

34. *1982 Directory: Investor-owned Hospitals and Hospital Management Companies* (Little Rock, Ark.: Federation of American Hospitals, 1981), p. 9.

35. "The Chain: A Survival Formula for Hospitals," *Business Week*, January 26, 1978, p. 113.

36. Vince DiPaolo, "AHS Studies Service Effectiveness," *Modern Health Care* 9 (May 1979):52.

37. H.S. Ruchlin, D.D. Pointer, and L.L. Cannedy, "A Comparison of For-profit Investor-owned Chain and Non-profit Hospitals," *Inquiry* 10 (December 1973):13–23.

38. Ann Hughey, "Health Care," *Forbes*, January 5, 1981, p. 32.

39. Rita Ricardo-Campbell, *The Economics of Politics of Health* (Chapel Hill: University of North Carolina Press, 1982), p. 78.

40. "As Controversy Mounts Over Hospitals-for-profit," *U.S. News and World Report*, December 10, 1984, p. 61.

41. Jennifer Bingham-Hull, "Hospital Chains Battle Health Insurers, But Will Quality Lose in the War?" *Wall Street Journal*, February 11, 1985, p. A-2.

42. See, for example, *Studies in the Comparative Performance of Investor-owned and Not-for-profit Hospitals*, four volumes (Washington, D.C.: Lewis and Associates, 1981).

43. "Veterans' Benefits Up for Cuts," *The Sun* (Baltimore), November 20, 1984, p. A-1.

44. Ibid., p. A-6.

45. "U.S. Creating Care Quotas for Hospitals," *The Sun* (Baltimore), July 29, 1984, p. A-13.

46. Ibid.

47. "Hospital Ratings Will Open to Public," *The Evening Sun* (Baltimore), April 16, 1985, p. A-14.

6
Medicaid

Medicaid is a combined federal and state program which results in the provision of medical assistance to certain categories of low income persons, including those on welfare and some of the medically indigent (persons whose incomes are too low to pay for medical care). The program is administered and roughly half the costs are absorbed by the state and local governments.

The history of joint federal–state health care programs goes back over thirty-five years. The Social Security Amendments of 1950 provided federal matching funds for medical payments to hospitals, physicians, and other providers of medical care on behalf of those receiving public assistance. By 1960, about forty states were participating in this program, with medical care expenditures reaching $0.5 billion. The Social Security Amendments of 1960, known as the Kerr–Mills Act, greatly increased federal assistance for health care. The proportion of federal funds was increased as coverage was provided to the medically indigent elderly who did not require cash assistance. In 1965 Medicaid replaced the Kerr–Mills Act and thus increased the level of benefits as well as the breadth of the program. The new legislation also tried to impose more uniformity on state programs.[1]

The framers of Medicaid legislation apparently gave little consideration to future costs. Medicaid continued the pattern of federal–state financing of medical care for the poor begun under the Kerr–Mills program. Under Medicaid, as under Kerr–Mills, the federal contribution was inversely related to state per capita income. The major difference between Kerr–Mills and Medicaid was an extension of mandatory eligibility and federal sharing to welfare recipients who were not aged, that is, to recipients of Aid to Families with Dependent Children (AFDC), whose health assistance had previously been a state responsibility. In addition, Medicaid provided an option for federal matching funds for care of the "medically needy" who were not eligible for welfare. Indeed, an original objective of Medicaid was to induce states to extend eligibility to all persons with income below a certain amount, regardless of whether or not they participated in the AFDC program. This early Medicaid objective was subsequently eliminated, resulting in a significant number of low-income persons becoming ineligible for Medicaid.

Medicaid, like Medicare, based reimbursement of providers on market prices or costs. State Medicaid programs were required to pay hospitals according to the Medicare cost-based standard. However, they were permitted to pay physicians at rates below Medicare reimbursement levels. Mandatory covered services (which could not be subject to copayment or deductible) included hospital care, physicians' services, diagnostic services, family planning advice, and nursing home care in skilled nursing facilities. Screening and treatment of children were subsequently added to the mandatory coverage category. Optional coverage items included services in intermediate care facilities, dental care, drugs, eyeglasses, and some other medical services. Cost sharing was eventually permitted for some of these optional services and for hospital and physicians' services provided to the medically indigent.[2]

Mandatory eligibility is now required for persons receiving cash assistance under federally funded transfer programs. Therefore, persons eligible for income transfers under AFDC are automatically eligible for Medicaid. States have considerable flexibility in establishing income levels or other conditions for AFDC eligibility, and are indirectly able to control the number of persons who qualify for Medicaid assistance. Persons who are mandatory recipients of Supplemental Security Income (SSI), a federal program for the aged, blind, or disabled, are also automatically eligible for Medicaid. The income limits for SSI are established by the federal government.

Optional beneficiaries are those for whom states may receive federal matching funds but whose coverage is not required by federal legislation. This group includes medically needy families with dependent children whose incomes are above the state AFDC limit, as well as elderly persons who do not qualify for cash assistance. Many of the latter have large medical or nursing home bills.

Since Medicaid eligibility is primarily tied to AFDC eligibility, the former program is subject to the limitations of the latter. While AFDC is limited in a majority of states to families without a father residing in the home, twenty-four states and two jurisdictions also extend AFDC and Medicaid coverage to families with unemployed fathers who are not receiving unemployment compensation. Seventeen states and three jurisdictions cover all children in families with income below AFDC eligibility level, regardless of the family composition or the employment status of the parents.

The thirty states covering the medically needy establish income, asset, and family-composition tests similar to those for public assistance recipients. Medically needy income levels for a family of four as of March 1983 ranged from $9,600 in California to $2,460 in Tennessee.[3] Under the so-called spend-down provision, families with incomes above these levels may also be eligible if their incomes are below this amount after deducting medical expenses incurred.

As a result of the complex set of eligibility requirements, the following low-income persons do not quality for Medicaid assistance.

1. Widows and other single persons under 65 and childless couples
2. Most two-parent families (which constitute 70 percent of the rural poor and almost half the poor families in metropolitan areas)
3. Families with a father working at a marginal, low-paying job
4. Families with an unemployed father in the twenty-six states that do not extend welfare payments to this group, and unemployed fathers receiving unemployment compensation in other states
5. Medically needy families in the twenty states that do not voluntarily provide this additional coverage
6. Single women pregnant with their first child in the twenty states that do not provide welfare aid or eligibility for the unborn child
7. Children of poor families not receiving AFDC in the thirty-three states that do not take advantage of the optional Medicaid category called "all needy children under 21"[4]

In 1983, an estimated 21.5 million people received services covered by Medicaid. This was the same number who received services in 1979. However, between 1979 and 1983 the number of people living in poverty rose from 25 million to nearly 35 million. Thus, only 55 to 60 percent of the poverty population was covered by Medicaid in 1983.[5]

Medicaid Costs

The cost of the Medicaid program has increased rapidly. Combined federal and state-local expenditures increased from $3.5 billion in 1968 to $35.6 billion in 1983. (See table 6–1).

Three factors explain almost all the increases in expenditures. These are the increase in the number of Medicaid recipients covered under the AFDC program; sustained medical care price inflation; and the high cost of skilled nursing facilities and intermediate care facilities for the aged, poor, and disabled. Expenditures for these two items more than doubled between 1973 and 1983.

The rapid growth in the number receiving welfare payments in the late 1960s and early 1970s accounted for a large portion of the increased cost of Medicaid. Between 1968 and 1972 the total number of Medicaid recipients rose by 70 percent. Since the economy was relatively prosperous at that time, most of the increase was due to the increased number of eligible people

Table 6–1

Number of Recipients, Total Payments, and Payments per Recipient under Medicaid, Fiscal Years 1968–1983

Fiscal Year	Number of Recipients (millions)	Total Federal and State Payments (billions)	Payments per Recipient	Medical Care Price Index 1968 = 100	Payments per Recipient in 1968 $
1968	11.5	$ 3.5	$ 300	100.0	$300
1969	12.1	4.4	361	106.9	338
1970	14.5	4.1	354	113.7	311
1971	18.0	6.4	356	121.0	297
1972	18.0	7.4	411	124.9	329
1973	19.6	8.6	440	129.8	339
1974	21.1	10.0	474	141.8	334
1975	22.2	12.3	554	158.9	348
1976	22.9	14.1	615	173.9	354
1977	22.9	16.3	710	192.9	368
1978	22.2	18.0	810	207.8	390
1979	21.5	20.5	953	228.0	418
1980	21.6	25.7	1,190	252.9	471
1981	22.1	30.4	1,376	280.2	491
1982	21.8	32.9	1,509	312.7	483
1983	21.5	35.6	1,656	342.0	484

Source: U.S. Department of Health, Education, and Welfare, Health Care Financing Administration, *Data on the Medicaid Program: Eligibility, Services, Expenditures, Fiscal Years 1966–1977* (Washington, D.C.: Institute for Medicaid Management, 1977), p. 34; Donald Muse and Darwin Sawyer, *The Medicare and Medicaid Data Book, 1981* (Washington, D.C.: U.S. Department of Health and Human Services, 1982), pp. 13, 20; Robert Gibson, Katherine Levit, Helen Lazenby, and Daniel Waldo, "National Health Expenditures, 1983," *Health Care Financing Review* 6, no. 2 (Winter 1984):20–21.

applying for benefits. Estimates indicate that the percentage of eligible people participating in AFDC increased from 60 percent to more than 90 percent.[6]

The second major factor is the sustained inflation in medical care prices. After the removal of wage and price controls on the health industry in April 1974, the medical care price index rose at an annual rate of 13 percent in sharp contrast with the rate of 4 percent when the economic stabilization program was in effect.[7] Hospital costs went up at the even faster annual rate of 16 percent. From 1975 to 1983 medical care prices rose an average of 10 percent annually, with the prices of hospital services rising slightly faster. These higher prices were reflected in increasing Medicaid expenditures.

Annual Medicaid payments per recipient in constant 1968 "medical dollars" (expenditures divided by the medical care price index) averaged $484 in 1983, as compared to $338 in 1969. (See table 6–1.) From 1969 to 1977, there was little growth in real per capita expenditures. However, since 1977, payments per recipient have risen rapidly, reflecting greater utilization.

The final source of expenditure increases under Medicaid is the high cost of institutionalization for the elderly, poor, and disabled population that is unable to carry out normal daily activities without nursing assistance. The aged are the only sizable group for which there has been any substantial increase in dollar expenditure in recent years. The increase was more than 30 percent between 1968 and 1980. The tendency to place large numbers of the elderly in nursing homes—where average Medicaid expenditures exceeded $8,000 a person in 1983—accounts for a major portion of Medicaid costs. More than two-thirds of Medicaid expenditures are for services to aged or disabled adults.[8]

Medicaid Recipients

The largest group of Medicaid recipients consists of dependent children under the age of 21. However, as indicated in table 6–2, this is the group that is least costly (per recipient) to serve. Dependent children and the adults in their families constitute 69 percent of Medicaid recipients, but are responsible for only about 26 percent of Medicaid expenditures. The largest share of

Table 6–2
Medicaid Recipients and Payments by Eligibility Category, Fiscal Year 1983

Basis of Eligibility	Recipients		Payments[a]		Average Payment per Recipient (dollars)
	Number (thousands)	Percentage of Total	Dollars (millions)	Percentage of Total	
Age 65 or over	3,247	15.1	11,954	37.0	3,682
Blindness	76	0.4	183	0.6	2,408
Permanent and total disability	2,956	13.8	11,183	34.6	3,783
Dependent children under age 21	9,418	43.8	3,822	11.8	406
Adults in families with dependent children	5,467	25.4	4,483	13.9	820
Other	1,325	6.2	725	2.2	547
Total	21,494[b]	100.0[b]	32,351[c]	100.0	1,505

Source: Unpublished tabulations provided by the Health Care Financing Administration.

[a]Payments are Medicaid vendor payments made to providers of service for care rendered to eligible individuals. Amounts include both state and federal share.

[b]Categories do not add to total because of a small number of recipients who are in more than one category during the year.

[c]Detail does not add to total because of rounding.

Medicaid payments—37.0 percent—is for services to the elderly, reflecting the cost of long-term nursing home services as well as the greater need for medical services within this age group. The disabled category, which includes terminally ill persons under age 65, the mentally retarded, and poor individuals with work-related disabilities, includes less than 14 percent of recipients, but accounts for about 35 percent of Medicaid payments.

Most of the recent increases in Medicaid payments have gone to the aged and disabled. From 1980 to 1983, 46 percent of the total growth in Medicaid payments was for disabled persons, and 36 percent was for other persons over age 65. Adults in families with dependent children is the only category of persons eligible for Medicaid in which the number of recipients has been rising. A significant source of growth in Medicaid payments for the disabled is the recent trend toward deinstitutionalization of the mentally retarded. The rate of growth in mentally retarded Medicaid recipients using intermediate care facilities (ICFs) has been greater than that for any other service. When the mentally retarded leave state institutions, they may become eligible for Medicaid benefits in ICFs or the community. The resulting increase in Medicaid expenditures comes from shifting costs away from state-funded institutions to the federal–state Medicaid program. In addition, this change frequently results in an upgrading from the largely custodial care of state institutions to the more rehabilitative care in Medicaid-funded ICFs.[9]

Although there has been appreciable aging of the nation's population, it has not affected the growth of Medicaid costs. In fact, the number of recipients over age 65 actually declined from 1980 to 1983.

There have been changes in utilization patterns by Medicaid hospital patients. The average length of stay has declined substantially, but this decline has been offset by an increase in the frequency of hospitalizations, which is far above the United States average. Physicians may have responded to pressure from professional standards review organizations (PSROs) to discharge their patients sooner, but Medicaid provides no incentive for physicians or their patients to seek alternatives to inpatient hospital services.

Medicaid payments for clinic services and home health services have been growing rapidly. However, they comprise only a small portion of Medicaid payments and account for only a small fraction of the recent increase in Medicaid expenditures. The rate of growth in payments for physicians' services, which have not involved cost-based reimbursement, has been much lower than the growth rates for other components. State limits on reimbursement amounts and the resulting decrease in the number of recipients using physicians' services (as physicians refuse to serve Medicaid patients) are contributing factors. Similarly, payments for (and use of) hospital outpatient services, which had previously grown rapidly, have recently been increasing more slowly, perhaps partly in response to the establishment of more restrictive reimbursement policies in some states.

Reducing the growth in Medicaid costs requires solving certain problems the program has in common with health insurance. Resolution of these issues will probably necessitate making Medicaid reimbursement mechanisms different from those for conventional insurance. Since recent growth in Medicaid costs has come mainly from inflation in medical care prices and increased use per recipient, these are the areas in which cost-savings efforts should focus. Reducing the growth in prices paid for services will require separating Medicaid from the third-party cost reimbursement system that has been a major factor in medical care price inflation. In addition, ways must be found to limit utilization by recipients. There is little evidence that Medicaid recipients have used services more than other persons with full insurance coverage, not does it appear that there is greater inefficiency in the provision of services under Medicaid than under other public or private programs. Cuts in Medicaid, therefore, would actually involve reductions in available services.[10]

Effect on Use and Health

A number of studies have clearly demonstrated that the Medicaid program improved the medical and dental care utilization of program participants.[11] In some cases, Medicaid beneficiaries used services about as frequently as middle- and upper-income people. A smaller fraction of those visits by Medicaid patients (as compared to the nonpoor), however, are to physicians in private offices, and relatively more occur in hospital outpatient departments. Considering the poor population alone, visit rates tend to be higher for those receiving Medicaid, but Medicaid recipients tend to be sicker than the poor as a whole. Davis and Reynolds suggest that the poor receiving public assistance (Medicaid-eligible) use physicians' services slightly more frequently than other persons.[12] But the non-Medicaid-eligible poor see physicians at a much lower rate than the poor in general.

Medicaid has reduced inequality in the use of physicians' services and has contributed to greater use of hospital care by the poor. However, there are still differences in use between the poor who are and are not Medicaid-eligible. Moreover, there is considerable difference in access to care among Medicaid patients, reflecting interstate differences in Medicaid requirements and benefits.

However, the effect of Medicaid on health is difficult to demonstrate. There have been substantial improvements in many health indicators since Medicaid legislation was passed in 1965, but the improvements are largely a continuation of earlier trends. Death rates from heart diseases, diabetes, and most other major causes (except lung cancer) have declined, but these trends began at least twenty years before the inception of Medicaid. Moreover, there is evidence that mortality is more directly related to income, education, and life style than to increased consumption of health services.[13] Since the research results available are not based on randomized experiments, it is not certain that self-selection in the use of medical services does not lead to an understatement of the effect of those services. The lack of a positive correlation between medical care and health may occur because causality moves in two opposite directions. In one, poor health results in greater use of medical care; and in the other, medical care improves health. That is, the effect of medical services on health may be obscured by the fact that persons with poor health need to use more medical services.

Since there are no aggregate data available on death rates by income class, attempts to examine health effects of the Medicaid program must use alternative measures for poverty in addition to imperfect measures of health. Since a higher proportion of nonwhites are poor, one such proxy measure is race. (This measure must be used cautiously since there may be racial effects that are independent of income.) A comparison of mortality by race and sex for the period 1965–1977 shows no clear pattern of differences by race. In addition, there is no other evidence that Medicaid has had a major effect on mortality rates for poor adults.

For infants, children, and others—particular targets of Medicaid and the Great Society programs that accompanied it—there is somewhat stronger evidence. The rates of fetal deaths, neonatal deaths, and maternal deaths all declined by larger percentages from 1965 to 1970 than in the preceding five years; and the decline was larger in absolute value and in percentage for blacks than for whites. The Medicaid program was likely a contributing factor, but the decline in fertility rates, particularly for women over thirty-five, may have also been important. In addition, the rapid gains in employment and income which occurred in the late 1960s may also have improved health.

Direct evidence of Medicaid's effect on the health of recipients is limited and conflicting. Friedman, Parker, and Lipworth found no effect of either Medicaid or private insurance on the rate of early diagnosis of breast cancer.[14] Kehrer and Wolin found no significant effect of Medicaid eligibility on birth weight of infants born to participants in the Gary income-maintenance experiments.[15] Grossman and Jacobowitz provide evidence that Medicaid coverage of first pregnancies accounts for about 7 percent of the reduction in neonatal mortality rates for nonwhites between 1964 and 1977, but their evidence suggests that such coverage is associated with higher neonatal mortality rates for whites.[16]

Thus, there are few improvements in health statistics that can be clearly attributed to Medicaid. However, this does not indicate that the Medicaid program has had no effect on health. The program probably has had positive effects even if they are difficult to measure. One must realize that it is always difficult to separate the effects of improved medical care on health from that of general socio-economic improvement.

The Distribution of Medicaid Benefits

Because Medicaid is a federal–state program that allows state governments considerable latitude in determining eligibility, the range and amount of Medicaid benefits, and reimbursement levels of health care providers, Medicaid benefits differ greatly from state to state.

Medicaid expenditures are concentrated in a few northern industrial states. In 1983, New York spent 19.4 percent of all Medicaid funds. California, with the second largest program, spent 11 percent. These two states, together with Michigan, Illinois, and Pennsylvania, accounted for 44 percent of total Medicaid expenditures.[17]

The state distribution of Medicaid funds does not correspond to the prevalence of poverty or sickness. The south, with approximately 45 percent of the nation's poor, receives 22 percent of all combined federal–state Medicaid funds.[18]

Differences between states arise because some states cover a greater fraction of their poor population and because some have more comprehensive benefits for eligible Medicaid recipients. Even for those covered by Medicaid, there are wide differences in benefit levels from state to state. Average payments per Medicaid recipient in fiscal 1983 ranged from $1,030 in Mississippi, to $2,632 in Nevada. The national figure was $1,505. The aged in Alabama receive services costing Medicaid an average of $1,612 per person, but in Pennsylvania, the cost is $5,065 per person.[19]

Part of the variation occurs because not all states cover the medically needy. However, even for welfare recipients, fiscal 1983 medical benefits per family eligible for AFDC averaged $742 in South Carolina and $1,698 in New York, though the national average was $1,048.[20] These differences would be of less importance if they actually reflected differences in medical care prices or statewide differences in morbidity. However, these are not the reasons for the differences. Benefit patterns are unrelated to health care needs or the costs of health and medical care.

For example, the average payment for physicians' services in fiscal 1983 was $491 in Alaska and $56 in Pennsylvania. In Oregon, 13 percent of the state's Medicaid recipients were hospitalized; in Texas and Tennessee, the figures were 25 and 27 percent, respectively. Iowa, Louisiana, and Maryland place few of their elderly in skilled nursing homes, but over half of the elderly Medicaid patients in Connecticut are in nursing homes. Average payments for skilled nursing facilities are $3,535 in Tennessee, but $11,545 in Connecticut. The national average is $8,051.[21]

Medicaid data show large differences in payments by race. The average payment on behalf of whites is about double the average payment for nonwhites.[22] Particularly discouraging is the fact that racial differences in average payment levels under Medicaid appear to be widening. Differences are most extreme in rural southern and western areas, where whites receive more than twice the benefits received by blacks.

Sizable differences also exist between Medicaid benefits in urban and rural areas. Anderson and others found that average Medicaid expenditures (and other minor sources of free care) were $76 per poor child in central cities, and $5 per poor child in rural areas. Urban–rural differences also exist for other age groups. Benefits for the elderly poor in central cities are twice as large as for those living in rural areas.[23]

Lower medical benefits for rural families to some degree reflect the urban bias of the program. Many of the rural poor simply cannot qualify for Medicaid because they are not included in the narrow eligibility categories established for welfare. For example, only 40 percent of low-income rural persons are elderly or members of single-parent families. The urban poor may also have greater Medicaid participation rates because they tend to be more informed about eligibility for assistance, and also there are more organized groups working on their behalf in urban areas.

The lower benefit levels of rural residents also reflect the lack of medical resources and the greater distance to health care facilities. In most states Medicaid will not pay for services provided by a nurse practitioner or physician assistant unless a physician is present when medical services are provided. Health professionals other than physicians have helped to increase the supply of health manpower in rural areas. However, their effectiveness has been limited by supervision requirements and lack of third-party reimbursement under Medicaid. In 1977, the Social Security Act was amended to provide for Medicare and Medicaid reimbursement of rural health clinics. This has helped to pay the salaries of physician assistants and nurse practitioners employed in the clinics.

Transportation is also a significant barrier to medical care in some rural areas. Without special programs to bring patients to medical services or medical services to patients, many of the rural poor, particularly the aged, are unable to obtain care even if their payment for care is nominal. This accounts in part for the higher death rate as well as the greater incidence of chronic conditions and more serious disabling conditions among rural as compared to urban people.[24]

Provider Reimbursement

In the late 1970s through 1980s, states tried to contain costs of the Medicaid program through the use of more stringent eligibility requirements, imposition of service cutbacks and limitations, tighter administrative controls, and postponement of increases in physician reimbursement. It became obvious that changes had to be made in Medicaid cost-based provider reimbursement incentives for hospitals and nursing homes which made little effort to contain rising costs. Moreover, Medicaid eligibility rules led physicians to institutionalize patients so that they could receive necessary services. A growing number of states are redesigning their Medicaid programs in ways that emphasize tighter management of the care delivered and provide less freedom for beneficiaries to select their own providers of care.

Under the Omnibus Budget Reconciliation Act of 1981, federal Medicaid grants to states were reduced by 3 percent in 1982, 4 percent in 1983, and 4.5 percent in 1984. The 1981 budget law also altered Medicaid's rules for eligibility, benefits, and payment. As a result, 750,000 beneficiaries became ineligible for Medicaid services with an estimated Medicaid saving of $3.9 billion from 1982 to 1985.[25]

The Act also modified the long-standing freedom-of-choice policy that gave individual Medicaid recipients the freedom to obtain services from any qualified provider. States may now enter into arrangements to purchase laboratory services or medical devices through competitive bids, establish a lock-in feature which restricts the choice of provider by the beneficiary to low-cost providers, or implement a primary care network or case management system. Congress also authorized the Department of Health and Human Services to waive requirements in the Social Security Act that discouraged or restricted coverage of home-based and community-based long-term care.

There are many variations on the primary care network (PCN) theme, but there are common characteristics as well. A network is composed of primary care physicians, typically family practitioners. The network doctors agree to serve as the patient's main point of contact with the medical care system. The primary care physician network is augmented by a panel of specialists. Patients are "locked in" to their primary care physicians who must approve all specialty referrals. Thus, to the extent that the PCN will not pay for those services rendered by nonparticipating providers, the Medicaid recipient's choice of providers is limited. Physicians are reimbursed on a capitation basis and are at financial risk for primary care and, in some instances, specialty care and hospital services.[26]

Spending for nursing home services is the largest and most rapidly growing component of national Medicaid outlays. Most state Medicaid programs have adopted various forms of prospective reimbursement where rates and rate increases are negotiated or determined by formulas prior to each new fiscal year. The prospective methods are either facility-specific negotiated rates or class rates based on facility type, size, and location. Some states use a combination of methods. There are only ten states that use traditional retrospective methods for Medicaid reimbursement of nursing homes.[27]

With respect to hospital reimbursement, by 1983 only twenty-six states (accounting for 23 percent of inpatient expenditures) still used cost-based reimbursement methods in regards to Medicaid patients. Some states, such as New Jersey and Georgia, are using experimental systems of prospective reimbursement based on diagnostic-related groupings. Most of the other states have tended toward facility-specific budget review, rate of increase control, and other forms of prospective rate setting.[28]

Because state Medicaid authorities have not had to accept customary fees since 1981, but can instead set Medicaid reimbursement payments at their discretion using a fee schedule, many states can reimburse physicians at rates considerably below Medicare reimbursement levels. The average Medicaid reimbursement for a visit to a physician is approximately 65 percent of the average charge for non-Medicaid patients. In this context, two relevant facts are important. First, many physicians refuse to accept Medicaid patients or greatly limit their Medicaid patient load, and the willingness to accept such patients is a positive function of the level of Medicaid payments.[29] Second, even though they are paid considerably less than the market price, many physicians still provide services to Medicaid patients. However, if Medicaid costs are cut by reducing physicians' fees further, access for the poor will decline because fewer physicians will accept Medicaid patients.

Attempting to save money by limiting payment to physicians for their services is an inefficient way to reduce program costs. Payments to physicians for their services constitute less than 10 percent of total Medicaid outlays. However, many other services are highly complementary to physician care, and the doctor controls the use of those services to a considerable degree. By restructuring fee schedules or encouraging prepaid group practices so that physicians are rewarded for lower hospital, nursing home, laboratory, or prescription drug costs, Medicaid cost savings may increase even if physicians are reimbursed at a higher level. For example, raising the reimbursement rate for surgery, if it is conducted in a less costly outpatient setting, may cause the surgeon to change the place at which surgery is performed, but it may also result in an increase in surgery provided.

With the passage of the 1972 amendments to the Social Security Act, there began a gradual but consistent trend toward paying less than actual cost to hospitals with above-average costs.[30] These reimbursement limits may have resulted in the transfer of costs for public patients to states and to insurance companies.

If the amount Medicaid will pay to hospitals is reduced through a prospective payment system, several responses can be expected. First, access by Medicaid patients is likely to be reduced. If legally permissible, some hospitals may refuse to accept public patients. Moreover, some reduction in quality or intensity of care may occur.

If hospitals are required to provide service when revenue is less than cost, they must make up the deficit. If they consume working capital, they will eventually be forced to shut down. Charging other patients higher prices for care may not be feasibile in an increasingly competitive environment and it is also inequitable.

If payments to providers should be further reduced, one possible improvement in Medicaid policy would be to permit beneficiaries to supplement Medicaid payments with personal payment. The beneficiary who must travel a great distance for care because a nearby physician is unwilling to accept Medicaid patients may be better off if permitted to make up the difference between the Medicaid payment and the doctor's normal charge. Presumably the restriction on supplementation by beneficiaries is intended to prevent beneficiaries from being overcharged. However, the supplementation policy seems to work reasonably well for Medicare. A beneficiary faced with the choice of being unable to obtain care at a zero out-of-pocket price or care that he or she prefers with a small payment required may prefer the latter.

Most studies of physician participation in Medicaid have focused on primary care physicians, but the poor also need access to specialists. One study examined Medicaid participation rates for a national sample of 2,291 private practice physicians in nine medical and surgical specialties. Four-fifths of the specialists treated at least some Medicaid patients, with an average case load of 11.2 percent Medicaid patients. This level of participation was similar to results obtained elsewhere for primary care physicians. According to the study findings, a 10 percent increase in the Medicaid reimbursement rate would raise specialist participation by 3 percent. Other factors encouraging specialist participation included faster claims processing, fewer limits on the quantity of services covered, and more generous eligibility criteria.[31]

Nearly 60 percent of all Medicaid patients treated in private physician practices receive services from doctors whose patient volume is composed of at least 30 percent Medicaid patients.[32] However, these physicians do not appear to be operating "Medicaid mills." For example, visit length in large Medicaid practices is similar to that of non-Medicaid physicians, while ancillary services do not appear to be excessive. Medicaid doctors generally earn less than other private physicians. However, the physicians with large Medicaid practices may be less able than other doctors. The former are more likely to be older, non-Board certified, and graduates of foreign medical schools.

Copayments

With the passage of the Social Security Amendments of 1972, states were empowered to impose "nominal" cost-sharing requirements on optional Medicaid services for cash-assistance recipients and on any services for the medically needy. The TEFRA Act of 1982 introduced major changes in cost-sharing arrangements. States may now impose a nominal deductible, coinsurance, or copayment plan upon both the categorically and medically needy for any service

Table 6–3
Copayments, Various Health Services, Selected State Medicaid
Programs, March 1983

State	Service	Copayment Amount
California	Drugs	$ 1.00
District of Columbia	Eyeglasses	2.00
Iowa	Dental	3.00
Kansas	Optometrist	0.50
Michigan	Hearing aid	3.00
Nevada	Dentures	3.00
North Carolina	Chiropractor	0.50
South Carolina	Podiatrist	1.00
South Dakota	Inpatient (per stay)	25.00
Wisconsin	Inpatient (mental illness, per stay)	75.00

Source: Compiled from Donald Muse, Robert Clinkscale, Sally McCue, Maureen Fisher, and Phillip Hyatt, "Analysis of State Medicaid Program Characteristics," mimeographed (La Jolla Management Corporation, Washington, D.C., December 1983), pp. 111–17.

offered under the state plan. (See table 6–3.) However, the legislation prohibits cost sharing on the following: services furnished to individuals under eighteen years of age, pregnancy-related services, services for certain institutionalized persons who must spend all their income for medical care (except for a personal needs allowance), emergency services, family-planning services, and services received by certain HMO enrollees.[33]

Early results of the Health Insurance Study by Newhouse show that copayments reduce expenditures on medical services. The effect of copayments has not varied with the income of the participating families. However, concern that small copayments would result in large reductions in use appear to be unfounded.[34]

Effect of Medicaid Cutbacks on Health— A Case Study of California

To control rising health costs, California enacted legislation in 1982 that eliminated Medicaid for its 270,000 medically indigent adults. Responsibility for providing care to this population was transferred to the counties on January 1, 1983.[35] Block grants made available by the state to the counties to provide health services for this population were approximately 70 percent of what the state would have spent had the Medicaid program for medically-indigent adults remained in effect. For medically needy adults whose usual source of care was not the county health system, the new policy meant that care was disrupted and relationships with previous physicians were terminated.

Six months after this policy had gone into effect the general health status of the medically indigent patients had worsened. For example, those with hypertension experienced a significant rise in their blood pressure after they were terminated from the Medicaid program. Only 50 percent of these individuals had a usual source of care six months after termination in comparison to 96 percent prior to termination. Only 60 percent of these persons were satisfied with their care in July 1983, while 91 percent were satisfied at the end of 1982. A comparison group of Medicaid enrollees who were unaffected by the Medicaid cutback in California experienced no decline in either health status, satisfaction with health care, or percentage with a usual source of care.[36]

Long-Term Care

The Medicaid program, designed to purchase health care for indigent Americans, has evolved into the primary purchaser of long-term care in the United States. Payments for these services also absorb the largest share of the Medicaid budget. Many factors are responsible for this evolution of Medicaid. Among the more important are the aging of the population, the rising cost of nursing home care, and federal Medicaid and Medicare policies. The Medicare program, which is the federal health insurance program for the elderly, will only reimburse a maximum of 100 days of care received at a skilled care facility in any one stay. Also, Medicare does not reimburse for services received at intermediate care facilities. Paradoxically, this places the major public burden of paying for long-term care on Medicaid—the health program for the poor—and not on Medicare—the health program for the elderly.[37]

Spending for nursing home care rose from 4.9 percent of total national health care spending in 1965, to 8.8 percent in 1981. The public sector has become the dominant purchaser of institutional long-term care, with its share of the total bill increasing from 34 percent in 1965, to 57 percent in 1981. Within the public sector, the federal share of this expense has been declining (from 65 percent of the public nursing home bill in 1965, to 54 percent in 1981) while state and local governments have accounted for a larger portion of the total (rising from 35 percent in 1965, to 46 percent in 1981).[38]

During 1973, private patients or their families paid 49 percent of the total cost for nursing home services. The Medicaid program paid 43 percent. At that time, Medicare paid only 2.5 percent of total nursing home costs, a percentage that has been declining since the mid-1970s. By 1975 the Medicaid program became the largest spender for nursing home services, and by 1980 it paid 50 percent of these expenditures.

Table 6–4 indicates the increasing share of the Medicaid budget accounted for by long-term care spending, particularly for intermediate care. Medicaid spending for intermediate care will rise from 18 percent of total Medicaid spending in 1975, to an estimated 29 percent in 1985. Medicaid payments for hospital care will decline slightly from 28 percent to an estimated 25 percent of total Medicaid spending over this period.

Table 6–5 presents the major Medicaid expenditure categories and the annual increases of each. The annual increases for Medicaid expenditures to intermediate care facilities are very large, averaging 21.4 percent per year between 1975 and 1985. To give perspective to these intermediate care cost increases, average annual cost increases between 1975 and 1985 are 13.5 percent for the total Medicaid program, 12.7 percent for hospital care, and 8.8 percent for skilled care. Given the fiscal problems facing most states and the cutbacks in federal Medicaid cost sharing, methods must be found to contain these rapidly increasing payments to intermediate care facilities if the state programs are to remain financially solvent. With payments to skilled and intermediate care facilities absorbing roughly 43 cents out of every Medicaid dollar during 1983, there is the strong possibility that nursing home expenditures will force cutbacks in other health services within Medicaid. Equally

Table 6–4
Major Medicaid Spending Categories
(in millions of dollars)

Year	Total Medicaid		Hospital		Skilled Care		Intermediate Care[a]	
1985[b]	40,762	(100)[c]	10,325	(25)[c]	5,389	(13)	11,975	(29)[c]
1984[b]	37,209	(100)	9,264	(25)	5,051	(14)	10,940	(29)
1983[b]	34,285	(100)	8,567	(25)	4,753	(14)	10,033	(29)
1982	29,906	(100)	7,822	(26)	4,383	(15)	8,587	(29)
1981	27,284	(100)	7,203	(26)	4,160	(15)	7,417	(27)
1980	23,301	(100)	6,271	(27)	3,709	(16)	6,198	(27)
1979	20,462	(100)	5,650	(28)	3,683	(18)	5,272	(26)
1978	17,975	(100)	4,988	(28)	3,097	(17)	4,285	(24)
1977	16,276	(100)	4,603	(28)	2,687	(17)	3,518	(22)
1976	14,135	(100)	3,938	(28)	2,488	(18)	2,791	(20)
1975	12,292	(100)	3,411	(28)	2,446	(20)	2,216	(18)

Source: Estimates for 1983, 1984, and 1985 were obtained from the U.S. Department of Health and Human Services, Health Care Financing Administration, Office of Financial and Actuarial Analysis. Data for 1975–1982 are from the U.S. Department of Health and Human Services, Health Care Financing Administration, Office of Policy, Planning, and Research, *Medicaid State Tables—Recipients, Payments, and Services, Fiscal Years 1975–1982.*

[a]Includes ICF-MR (intermediate care facilities-mentally retarded).

[b]Figures are estimates.

[c]Figures in parentheses are percentages of total spending.

Table 6–5
Major Medicaid Spending Categories and Annual Cost Increases, 1975–1985

Year	Medicaid (millions)	Annual Increase (%)	General Hospital (millions)	Annual Increase (%)	Skilled Care (millions)	Annual Increase (%)	Intermediate Care[a] (millions)	Annual Increase (%)
1985[b]	$40,762	9.5	$10,325	11.5	$5,389	6.7	$11,975	9.5
1984[b]	37,209	8.5	9,264	8.1	5,051	6.3	10,940	9.0
1983[b]	34,285	14.6	8,567	9.5	4,753	8.4	10,033	16.8
1982	29,906	9.6	7,822	8.6	4,383	5.4	8,587	15.8
1981	27,284	17.1	7,203	14.9	4,160	12.2	7,417	19.7
1980	23,301	13.9	6,271	11.0	3,709	10.1	6,198	17.6
1979	20,462	13.8	5,650	13.3	3,368	8.8	5,272	23.0
1978	17,975	10.4	4,988	8.4	3,097	15.3	4,285	21.8
1977	16,276	15.1	4,603	16.9	2,687	8.0	3,518	26.0
1976	14,135	15.0	3,938	15.5	2,488	0.9	2,791	25.9
1975	12,292	—	3,411	—	2,466	—	2,216	—
Average annual % increase, 1975–1985		13.6		12.7		8.8		21.4

Source: Estimates for 1983, 1984, and 1985 were obtained from the U.S. Department of Health and Human Services, Health Care Financing Administration, Office of Financial and Actuarial Analysis. Data for 1975–1982 are from the U.S. Department of Health and Human Services, Health Care Financing Administration, Office of Policy, Planning, and Research, *Medicaid State Tables—Recipients, Payments, and Services, Fiscal Years 1975–1982.*

[a]Includes intermediate care facilities-mentally retarded.
[b]Figures are estimates.

important, the quality of all health services provided for medicaid patients could deteriorate because of the Medicaid fiscal problems. If the program is to remain financially solvent, state Medicaid programs must reform long-term care reimbursement methods to contain rising costs.

From 1975 to 1982, state Medicaid programs using the prospective rate-setting mechanism consistently paid lower average per diem rates to skilled care and intermediate care facilities than did states using the retrospective method. Although these payment differences were not always statistically significant, the prospective mechanism was always associated with lower per diem reimbursement rates. Between 1975 and 1982, the average rate paid for skilled care in prospective payment states increased 89.9 percent, whereas the rate for retrospective states increased 120 percent. During this period the average Medicaid rate for intermediate care reimbursed with the prospective method increased 79.2 percent, whereas the Medicaid rate set with a retrospective mechanism increased 120 percent.

The prospective method of reimbursement does not appear to adversely affect the access of Medicaid patients to nursing home care. Indeed, the opposite results were observed. States using prospective rate setting consistently had the highest levels of utilization for both skilled and intermediate care. In fact, there is a pronounced trend toward declining access to skilled care by Medicaid recipients in states using the retrospective mechanism, but stable utilization patterns in states making use of prospective payments.

Many factors, other than the reimbursement mechanism, have an impact on the cost of long-term care to state Medicaid programs. Among the more important factors are wage rates paid in health facilities, the overall cost of living, and even the political climate of the states. Difference among the states in wage rates for licensed practical nurses, for example, explains as much as 82.6 percent of the variance in Medicaid per diem rates for skilled care. Linked to wage rates is the cost of living. Difference among states in living costs explains as much as 59.8 percent of the variance in Medicaid payments to intermediate care facilities.[39]

Medicaid Reform

Proposals for Medicaid reform can be classified into three broad categories: to alter the eligibility criteria and coverage of the poor, to reduce Medicaid benefits, and to change the federal role. The optimal federal role is highly debatable.

For example, a shift in federal policy might involve eliminating matching federal grants and substituting block grants to the states. Those who advocate block grants maintain that they give the states greater flexibility in deciding how to use Medicaid funds. One disadvantage of block grants is that they might encourage Medicaid recipients to migrate from states with meager benefits to states with high benefit levels. However, the degree of responsiveness of migration rates to Medicaid benefit levels is unknown.

Another policy alternative is to tie the federal contribution to a program of basic Medicaid benefits considered essential in all states. Those states who desired to supplement these basic benefit levels would be required to do so with their own funds.[40] A third option is to steadily reduce the federal contribution to Medicaid by a fixed percentage. This was the policy used by the Reagan administration under the Omnibus Budget Reconciliation Act of 1981.

One way to limit Medicaid hospital costs is to contract with selected hospitals on a competitive bid basis. California is experimenting with this program. Arizona is conducting a demonstration of a different approach to providing Medicaid services. Nearly all recipients must choose between prepaid organizations that are reimbursed on a capitation basis. All care must be provided or authorized by the health care organization which also is at financial risk for the provision of health services. This system is similar to the HMOs which many employees choose under their private health insurance plan options.

Alternatives to Long-Term Care under Medicaid

Long-term care under Medicaid must confront different problems. The major issue is the growth in demand for long-term care caused by the aging of the population. The elderly population doubled between 1950 and 1980 and will double again by 2030, reaching one-fifth of the total U.S. population.[41]

Because institutional care is very expensive, one alternative to long-term care under Medicaid is less costly community care for the elderly. This could involve adult day care, paid providers of home care, as well as informal support by family members. A related proposal is to give families tax credits or deductions if they maintain severely disabled family members at home rather than placing them in a nursing home or intermediate care facility.

Another approach is to emphasize private voluntary financing mechanisms for long-term care. One of these is the life-care contract in which the elderly individual is guaranteed lifetime care in a setting that combines residential living with specialized long-term care services. The participant pays a lump sum enrollment charge and, afterwards, monthly fees. This arrangement represents a capitated approach where the provider is at risk. The provider is at risk because if many individuals incur high medical charges the owners of the facility will incur a financial loss. Thus management has an incentive to provide cost-effective services including alternatives to institutional care.

Summary

Medicaid is a combined federal–state program which provides medical assistance to about two-thirds of all low-income persons. Because of state differences in eligibility criteria and access to providers, Medicaid benefits are concentrated in a small number of northern industrial states. California, which used to have a generous Medicaid program, has become increasingly restrictive.

The rapid increase in Medicaid costs, which reflects both medical care price inflation and higher utilization, has caused both state and federal government, to impose budget cutbacks and a variety of cost-containment measures. In many states, hospitals and nursing homes are no longer reimbursed on a retrospective cost basis, but on the basis of prospective costs. Reimbursement rates for physicians are being scaled back in relative terms and many states are restricting the beneficiary's freedom of choice of provider in order to encourage patients to utilize certain low-cost providers. This may reduce the willingness of some physicians to accept Medicaid patients.

Because of recent legislation, states are able to impose copayments on a greater variety of health services under Medicaid. This may deter utilization and worsen health.

In California, the elimination of the medically needy from Medicaid eligibility has resulted in a lower health status for these persons. Those whose eligibility was unaffected, however, experienced no change in health status or satisfaction with care.

Several proposals to reform Medicaid were discussed. Block grants are advocated by those who desire more flexibility for state programs, but differences in state benefit levels could encourage interstate migration. State contracts with selected hospitals on a competitive bid basis may slow down the growth in Medicaid expenditures.

Long-term care under Medicaid is becoming an increasing problem due to the aging population. Programs which emphasize home care may be more cost-effective than present reliance on institutional settings.

Notes

1. Karen Davis and Cathy Schoen, *Health and the War on Poverty: A Ten Year Appraisal* (Washington, D.C.: The Brookings Institution, 1978), p. 51.

2. Robert Stevens and Rosemary Stevens, *Welfare Medicine in America: A Case Study of Medicaid* (New York: Free Press, 1974), pp. 156–160 and 282–299.

3. Donald Muse, "Analysis of State Medicaid Program Characteristics," mimeographed (La Jolla Management Corporation, December 1983), p. 39.

4. Davis and Schoen, op. cit., p. 53.

5. Health Care Financing Administration, "Medicaid Recipients by Maintenance Assistance Status and by HHS Region and State: Fiscal Year 1983," unpublished tabulation.

6. John Palmer, "Government Growth in Perspective," *Challenge*, 19, no. 2 (May–June 1976):43.

7. U.S. Department of Health, Education, and Welfare, Office of Research and Statistics, *Medical Care Expenditures, Prices, and Costs: Background Book*, DHEW Publication No. (SSA)75-11909 (Washington, D.C.: U.S. Government Printing Office, 1976), p. 22.

8. Health Care Financing Administration, op. cit.

9. Thomas Grannemann and Mark Pauly, *Controlling Medicaid Costs* (Washington, D.C.: American Enterprise Institute for Public Policy Research, 1982), p. 11.

10. Ibid., p. 14.

11. See, for example, Karen Davis and Roger Reynolds, "The Impact of Medicare and Medicaid on Access to Medical Care," in Richard Rosett, ed., *The Role of Health Insurance in the Health Services Sector* (New York: Neale Watson Academic Publications for the National Bureau of Economic Research, 1976), p. 404; Margaret Olendzki, Richard Grann, and Charles Goodrich, "The Impact on Medicaid on Private Care for the Urban Poor," *Medical Care* 10, no. 3 (May–June 1972):204; Dennis Leverett and Anthony Jong, "Variations in Use of Dental Care Facilities by Low-Income White and Black Urban Populations," *Journal of the American Dental Association* 80, no. 1 (January 1970):139.

12. Davis and Reynolds, op. cit.

13. See Victor Fuchs, *Who Shall Live? Health, Economics, and Social Choice* (New York: Basic Books, 1974), chaps. 1–2; Joseph Newhouse and Lindy Friedlonder, "The Relationship Between Medical Resources and Measures of Health," *Journal of Human Resources* 15, no. 2 (Spring 1980):200–18.

14. Bernard Friedman, Paul Parker, and Leslie Lipworth, "The Influence of Medicaid and Private Health Insurance on the Early Diagnosis of Breast Cancer," *Medical Care* 1 (November–December 1973):485–90.

15. Barbara Kehrer and Charles Wolin, "Impact of Income Maintenance on Low Birth Weight: Evidence from the Gary Experiment," *Journal of Human Resources* 14, no. 4 (Fall 1979):434–62.

16. Michael Grossman and Stephen Jacobowitz, "Variations in Infant Mortality Rates among Counties of the United States: The Roles of Public Policies and Programs," *Demography* 18, no. 4 (November 1981):708, 710.

17. Health Care Financing Administration, "Medicaid Recipients by Maintenance Assistance Status and by HHS Region and State: Fiscal Year, 1983," unpublished tabulation.

18. Ibid.

19. Ibid.

20. Ibid.

21. Ibid.

22. Donald Muse and Darwin Sawyer, *The Medicare and Medicaid Data Book, 1981* (Washington, D.C.: U.S. Department of Health and Human Services, 1982), pp. 19, 25.

23. Ronald Andersen, Joanna Kravits, Odin Anderson, and Joan Daley, *Expenditures for Personal Health Services: National Trends and Variations, 1953–1970*, DHEW Publication No. (HRA) 74-3105 (Washington, D.C.: U.S. Department of Health, Education, and Welfare, Health Resources Administration, 1973), p. 52.

24. Davis and Schoen, op. cit., pp. 81–82.

25. John Inglehart, "Medicaid in Transition," *New England Journal of Medicine* 309, no. 14 (October 6, 1983):868–69.

26. John Inglehart, "Medicaid Turns to Prepaid Managed Care," *New England Journal of Medicine* 308, no. 16 (April 21, 1983):978.

27. Muse et al., p. 123.

28. Ibid., p. 137.

29. Frank Sloan, Janet Mitchell, and Jerry Cromwell, "Physician Participation in State Medicaid Programs," *Journal of Human Resources* 13, supplement (1978): 211–45.

30. Public Law 92-603, section 223, excludes from the definition of reasonable cost "any part of incurred cost found to be unnecessary in the efficient delivery of needed health services." The open-endedness of this provision has led some to suggest it as a possible means of sharply reducing payments to hospitals without the need for further legislation.

31. Janet Mitchell, "Medicaid Participation by Medical and Surgical Specialists," *Medical Care* 21, no. 9 (September 1983):929.

32. Council of Economic Advisors, *Economic Report of the President* (Washington, D.C.: U.S. Government Printing Office, 1985), p. 155.

33. Muse et al., p. 110.

34. Joseph Newhouse et al., "Some Interim Results from a Controlled Trial of Cost Sharing in Health Insurance," *New England Journal of Medicine* 305, no. 25 (December 17, 1981):1501–07.

35. Nicole Lurie, Nancy Ward, Martin Shapiro, and Robert Brook, "Termination from Medi-Cal—Does It Affect Health?" *New England Journal of Medicine* 311, no. 7 (August 16, 1984):480–81.

36. Ibid., pp. 482–83.

37. Robert Buchanan, "Medicaid Cost Containment: Prospective Reimbursement for Long-Term Care," *Inquiry* 20 (Winter 1983):334–42.

38. Mark Freeland and Carol Schender, "National Health Expenditures: Short-Term Outlook and Long-Term Projections," *Health Care Financing Review* 2 (Winter 1981):97–138.

39. Buchanan, op. cit., p. 342.

40. Council of Economic Advisors, op. cit., p. 156.

41. Ibid., p. 157.

7

Health Maintenance Organizations

The health maintenance organization (HMO) is not a new concept in health care. They have been in existence since the late 1920s, but were then called prepaid group practice plans or foundations for medical care.

HMOs are integrated organizations of various health providers responsible for providing and overseeing the comprehensive health care of their enrollees. In the fee-for-service system, the physician rarely coordinates total patient care, particularly if the patient is referred elsewhere. The centralization of records, continuity of care, and overall responsibility assumed by the HMO theoretically makes for superior care and more satisfied patients.

A second basic feature of HMOs is the capitation payment made by the enrollee to the HMO. Since the HMO is at risk for health care costs, it has a strong incentive to reduce utilization, especially for high-cost services such as inpatient hospital care. Simultaneously, there is an incentive to encourage and to provide preventive services that are cost-effective in the long run. (It is usually assumed that preventive care is less costly than curative care.) Similarly, early detection in many instances will reduce total treatment costs.

Although all HMOs take on risk through a capitation payment for some segment of health care, they differ in three ways: the method of payment to their physicians, the amount of care for which they are at risk, and the organization and delivery of services.[1] Different economic incentives are theoretically operating with each of these variations, resulting in different outcomes.

The increasing popularity of HMOs is based on several assumptions about their differences from the traditional fee-for-service system: (1) lower hospital utilization and subsequent lower costs; (2) continuity of care rather than fragmentation; (3) emphasis on prevention, with early detection and treatment, rather than emphasis on acute care; (4) increased accessibility to and use of primary medical care; and (5) greater satisfaction with medical care received.[2]

HMO Models

The predominant and traditional HMO structure is organized as a group practice plan in which physicians are salaried. The HMO is at risk for most care including hospitalization. Primary care is provided in a multispecialty clinic setting often linked to the HMO's own hospital. This model should have the lowest hospitalization and surgery rates and should place greatest emphasis on preventive care as compared to other approaches for several reasons.

1. Since hospitalization is the most costly form of care, the HMO would be expected to institute control mechanisms to keep utilization to a minimum.

2. Salaried physicians do not gain financially by hospitalizing patients. Fee-for-service physicians, in contrast, have considerable financial incentive to hospitalize patients since they have briefer encounters with hospitalized patients than with those seen in their offices and, thus, their income per unit of time is greater in the hospital setting. Fee-for-service surgeons have considerable incentives for performing operations. Their income is totally dependent on the number and complexity of operations performed. However, salaried surgeons are paid the same amount regardless of the quantity of services provided. Moreover, the complexity of the surgery completed does not affect their income.

3. The organization of physicians in large multispecialty groups may also be responsible for limiting hospital use. Economies of scale allow for a wide variety of diagnostic procedures and treatment services to be provided on an outpatient basis, and back-up coverage on evenings and weekends eliminates the incentive for physicians to have patients hospitalized instead of providing services at the office. In addition, the peer pressure that results when physicians practice within the same organization may help avoid overutilization.

4. This organized setting would be expected to provide greater continuity and accessibility to care than the traditional solo practice. Most services, regardless of specialty, would be available to the HMO patient in the same physical location and usually at the same time. Referrals are within the organization rather than to a separate facility.

In addition to the group model HMO, there is the individual practice association (IPA) model which typically involves an HMO acting as a health plan which then contracts through an intermediary organization with independent office-based physicians to provide services. These physicians agree to accept payment by the HMO as payment in full and to allow a withholding of these fees which are placed at risk. The withheld fee is given the provider only if the HMO meets its financial goals. Thus, while the individual physician can increase his income by providing more services, he or she can lose money if the physicians collectively overtreat patients or order too many expensive tests.

The implications of various economic incentives on the supply of services by the HMO and its providers are quite complex. When the physicians are salaried and share in the financial success of the plan, they will both individually and as a group try to reduce utilization. When physicians are paid on a fee-for-service basis within a group or IPA-type HMO, this incentive to expand utilization will be only partially offset by the collective risk sharing. This is especially true in IPAs in which the prepaid patients typically account for less than 15 percent of the physician's total caseload.[3]

To counteract the reduced incentive to limit utilization, IPAs have organized peer-review processes with predetermined standards of use against which physicians' practices are compared. Some early success of this type of peer review has been reported, but the concept is relatively new and relatively untested.[4]

HMO Legislation

In February 1971, President Richard Nixon delivered a health message to Congress in which he called for innovation and reform in the delivery of health care to slow down the rapid increase in health care costs. He advocated expansion of the health maintenance organization (HMO) concept.[5]

In 1973, Public Law 93-222 was passed by Congress. That act provided federal funding for HMO development, relief from certain restrictive state laws, and mandatory market access for HMOs.[6] For example, under the act certain classes of employers were required to give their employees the option of joining an HMO if one was available. To obtain this federal funding, the HMO had to conform to a strict and extensive set of requirements. Among these were: acceptance of community rating (a premium-setting concept where the high- and low-risk groups in a community are averaged); open enrollment (a concept of recruitment designed to guard against preferential selection of low-risk groups to the disadvantage of high-risk groups); and the provision of a mandatory set of basic benefits provided by the HMO.

Partly because of the slow growth of HMOs, the 1973 law was amended in 1976 by Public Law 94-460. The amendments had the effect of limiting the original restrictions, particularly with respect to open enrollment, community rating, and basic benefits. These changes were expected to increase the number of qualified HMOs. From the HMO perspective, meeting federal standards provided two distinct benefits—availability of federal loans and mandatory access to consumers—but the price for these benefits was federal regulation. Many HMOs declined to accept the federal standards. Some rejected these regulations because they could develop successfully without government benefits and preferred not being subject to the federal rules. The act was further amended in 1978 to provide loans for construction, training for managers, and safeguards against various financial abuses. The growth in number of HMOs and their enrollment has continued rapidly even though the government ended its loans and grant assistance programs in 1981 and 1982.

Number of HMOs and Enrollees

The Ross–Loos Clinic, founded in 1929, is generally accepted to be the first HMO. The number of HMOs grew slowly until 1965, at which time about twenty plans were in existence. By the beginning of 1970, the number had increased to twenty-six, with subsequent rapid acceleration. After 1970, the average rate of increase was about twenty to twenty-five HMOs per year.

Number of Health Maintenance Organizations United States, 1970–1984[7]

Year	Number of HMOs
1970	26
1972	35
1974	120
1976	160
1978	170
1980	230
1983	280
1984	300

The increased rate of growth starting at roughly the time of federal involvement in 1971 was not greatly affected by the passage of the HMO Act of 1973 and subsequent amendments to that law.

Prior to 1950, enrollment gains followed the slow but steady growth in the number of HMOs. In each of the next ten years, however, HMO enrollment more than doubled, reaching 3.1 million enrollees in the twenty-six prepaid plans in existence during 1970. In 1973, the year Congress passed the HMO Act, total enrollment was 4.4 million. Eleven years later the figure was 15.0 million or 6.6 percent of the total U.S. population.[8]

Why Are HMOs Increasing So Rapidly Now?

Employers are increasingly establishing higher deductibles and copayments in their conventional health insurance plans and employees are responding by electing HMO coverage. Moreover, independent physicians are raising charges in order to maintain income in the face of a declining number of patient visits. Consumers are more likely to drop their personal physicians when continued use of conventional insurance plans means higher costs. Doctor–patient relationships are likely not as strong as traditionally believed.

National HMOs

One sign of intensifying competition among HMOs is the development of a movement to create national HMOs by linking up independent HMOs with

Table 7-1
Multistate HMO Companies

Name	Total Enrollment 1983	Total Enrollment 1973	Number of Plans	Ownership
Kaiser–Permanente	4,389,000	2,651,389	9	Independent nonprofit
Blue Cross/Blue Shield Association (Chicago, Ill.)	1,300,000	256,000	58	Local Blue Cross/Blue Shield plans
Health Insurance Plan of Greater New York	875,000	757,628	2	Independent nonprofit
CIGNA Health Plan, Inc.	650,000	Founded 1978	8	CIGNA Corp.
Health America Corp.	394,842	Founded 1981	20	Stock company (OTC)
Pru Care, Inc.	340,000	Founded 1975	10	Prudential Insurance Co.
Maxicare Health Plans, Inc.	288,000	1,835	5	Stock company (OTC)
United States Health Care Systems, Inc.	211,000	Founded 1976	3	Stock company (OTC)
United Health Care Corp.	194,300	Founded 1977	8	Will offer stock
Med Centers Health Care, Inc.	169,134	1,000	4	Independent nonprofit
FHP, Inc.	149,000	40,000	3	Independent nonprofit
Share Development Corp.	80,000	Founded 1974	3	Privately held
Hancock–Dikewood Corp.	70,000	Founded 1980	4	John Hancock
Peak Health Care, Inc.	37,000	Founded 1979	3	Stock company (OTC)

Source: Compiled from "HMOs: A Decade of Growth," *Business Insurance*, December 19, 1983, p. 4.

other independent plans confined to one city or one metropolitan area. The Health Insurance Plan of New York (HIP), which has about 875,000 members, is not only one of the oldest HMOs, but is also the largest one concentrated in a single metropolitan area. Formerly confined to New York City and Long Island, HIP has recently opened its first physician office building in Westchester County, north of New York City.[9]

At present there are fourteen national HMO companies that own or manage 140 or about half the nation's HMOs. These fourteen companies serve about 9.2 million people, more than 60 percent of all the people enrolled in HMOs. (See table 7–1.)

The Effects of HMOs on Health Care Utilization

The literature evaluating the effects of health maintenance organizations in terms of their health services utilization, costs, and quality is extensive.[10] The major findings are:

1. Total costs (premium and out-of-pocket) for HMO enrollees are 10 to 40 percent lower than those for comparable people with conventional health insurance.

2. The rates of change in HMO costs per unit of service are not significantly different from cost increases incurred by other health care providers.

3. Enrollees in HMOs have about as many ambulatory visits as non-enrollees of similar socio-economic background.

4. Most of the HMO savings in medical costs are attributable to hospitalization rates, which are about 30 percent lower than those of conventionally insured populations.

5. The lower HMO hospitalization rates are due almost entirely to lower admission rates. The average length of stay does not differ from that of conventionally insured populations.

6. There is no evidence that discretionary or unnecessary medical utilization is greatly reduced by enrolling in HMOs.

7. Some critics of HMOs have argued that the lower costs of HMOs compared to a conventional fee-for-service setting is due to lower quality care. However, no methodologically sound study confirms this allegation. In fact, there is some evidence that HMOs provide higher quality care.[11]

The probable impacts of the differences in price, accessibility, and practice styles on utilization of services in different settings are summarized in table 7–2. It is not always clear whether increased or decreased utilization has a positive effect on health status. In general, increased access for patient-initiated visits is probably good, but that is not always the case. For instance, annual physical examinations for certain population groups are not cost-effective.[12] Moreover, frequent testing of healthy people increases the likelihood of false-positive results and subsequent anxiety, invasive testing, and iatrogenesis.

The various factors listed in table 7–2 influence utilization in different ways. Some variables such as net price, travel time and costs, and waiting time affect the consumer's demand function for medical services. Because IPA-HMOs involve physicians primarily in fee-for-service office-based practice, the only difference perceived by their HMO patients relative to the latter is the more comprehensive coverage of IPA-HMOs. The resulting lower net price will tend to increase utilization for the HMO patients. Prepaid group practice (PGP) patients also face a lower (or zero) net money price, but other factors change at the same time. They may not have a close relationship to a physician in the plan and, thus, are less likely to take the initial steps to obtain treatment. PGPs are usually centralized so that for most patients a longer trip will be involved in obtaining care. The PGP also frequently involves a different set of time costs. For example, appointments must be scheduled longer ahead of time, but once made, waiting time in the office is often shorter.[13] Thus, while fees are not used by HMOs as a rationing device to affect demand, as is the case for non-HMO patients, there are other differences associated with care provided by a group practice that make access both easier and more difficult to obtain.

HMO members are somewhat more likely than people with standard health insurance to see a physician at least once a year, yet among those utilizing services, HMO enrollees have somewhat fewer office visits and substantially fewer hospitalizations than non-HMO persons.[14]

This discussion may have suggested that the capitation or risk-sharing incentives of the HMO lead their physicians to directly change their patterns of practice. In fact, it is extremely unlikely that HMO physicians think about the economic aspects of their work each time they diagnose or treat a patient. Instead, certain routine practice patterns become habitual that are responsive to their economic incentives.

The situation in IPA and PGP-HMOs differs considerably. While definitive research has not been completed, it is unlikely that most physicians use different practice patterns for their fee-for-service and prepaid patients. The existing evidence indicates that both types of patient receive similar treatment in IPA-HMOs.[15] However, IPAs do exercise controls on patient care through hospital-based utilization review and through educational efforts to change general practice patterns by demonstrating that certain less costly techniques are equally effective.

Table 7-2
Probable Effects on Utilization of Services of Various Factors in Different Practice Settings

Type of Medical Care	Conventional Fee-for-Service and Insurance	IPA-HMOs: Fee-for-Service Practitioners at Risk	PGP-HMOs
Patient-Initiated Visits			
Price to consumer	− Initial and preventive visits often not covered	+ Comprehensive coverage of all visits	+ Comprehensive coverage of all visits
Knowledge of provider	+ Often a local physician with a longstanding relationship	+ Often a local physician with a longstanding relationship	− Often a local physician with no prior relationship with patient
Appointment lag	+ Typically short, urgent visits squeezed in	+ Typically short, urgent visits squeezed in	− Typically long, urgent visits routed to separate clinic
Accessibility to provider	+ Decentralized, likely close to patient	+ Decentralized, likely close to patient	− Centralized, generally further from patient
Waiting time in office	− Variable, often long because patients are squeezed in	− Variable, often long because patients are squeezed in	+ Typically short if appointment made in advance
Physician-Initiated Visits			
Physician incentives	+ Follow-up increases revenue	+/− Follow-up increases revenue more than risk sharing	− Follow-up reduces net income; substitute call-backs
Physician-Initiated Referral			
Physician incentives	+ Reciprocal referrals among different specialists encouraged by professional network, discouraged by prohibitions on fee splitting	+/− Referrals encouraged by professional network but discouraged by risk sharing	− Referral an attractive way to dump a problem patient, but collegial + financial costs if frequent
Price to consumer	+/− More likely covered than initial visit, still not complete coverage	+ Comprehensive coverage of all visits	+ Comprehensive coverage of all visits

Accessibility to provider	– Typically at a different location	– Typically at a different location	+ Centralized one-stop care
Incentives to return patient to primary care	+ Depends on nature of referral network	+ / – Depends on referral network, sometimes encouraged by HMO	– Typically encouraged by the system
Hospitalization			
Price to patient	– Often fairly comprehensive coverage but some copayments	+ Comprehensive coverage pays in full	+ Comprehensive coverage pays in full
Incentives for physician	+ Hourly income higher in hospital	+ / – Hourly income higher, but risk sharing tends to counter	– No additional income, costs are borne by plan

Source: Adapted from Harold Luft, "Health Maintenance Organizations and the Rationing of Medical Care," *Milbank Memorial Fund Quarterly/ Health and Society* 60, no. 2 (1982):276–77.

+ = tends to increase utilization.   – = tends to decrease utilization.   + / – = mixed or uncertain effects.

PGP physicians typically see only HMO patients. Thus any alteration of practice patterns is easier because a "two-class" system is unnecessary.

Allocation of Consumers among Systems

HMOs, like other insurers, obtain most of their members through groups of employees. Generally, only a small group of people are allowed to enroll as individual members and their premiums are frequently higher.

If an HMO wishes to enroll a certain kind of person (for example, the young and healthy), this may be accomplished in two ways. The first involves careful selection of the employee groups to whom the HMO enrollment option will be offered. For instance, firms with predominantly white-collar workers might be given high priority for enrollment, while blue-collar organizations would receive a lower priority.

The second strategy for selection would be to attract certain kinds of people within the employee group. Various approaches can be used to influence enrollment. Premiums are often set so that family coverage is relatively less expensive than individual coverage. This tends to attract families with children because of the lower per capita cost compared to individuals or two-person families. (This approach is also used by conventional insurers.) Moreover, HMOs have typically offered comprehensive coverage of maternity care, again making enrollment attractive for young, relatively healthy families.

The single most important determinant of whether someone will, given the option, choose a prepaid group practice is whether or not that person already has a personal physician. People with close or longstanding relationships with a personal physician tend not to join HMOs, while those without such ties are much more likely to join a prepaid plan.[16] One explanation for the absence of a strong physician-patient relationship is the lack of demand for medical care. Prepaid group practices not only attract people without strong physician ties but do not foster such a relationship. These two factors both lead to reduced utilization of services.[17]

Because the typical IPA-model HMO utilizes the facilities of many independent practitioners, it has less control than the PGP over some aspects of its delivery system, but it has greater control over others. For example, IPAs occasionally drop physicians from the HMO because of excessive utilization.

Clearly, it is in the plan's interest not to enroll those people who are above-average users of costly services. This not only benefits the plan, but the relatively low-cost people who do enroll receive comprehensive coverage and superior service at reduced average cost because, in part, the higher-cost individuals are excluded from the HMO.

This leads to a consideration of the environment in which HMOs exist. The notion of setting insurance premiums by community rating whereby all persons in a locale pay the same premium has been almost universally replaced by experience ratings in which firms with young, healthy employees pay lower premiums while those with older employees with concomitant higher health costs have higher premiums. HMOs generally used community ratings long before the HMO Act required it. Only recently, in the Omnibus Reconciliation Act of 1981, has the law been changed to allow HMOs to take into account differences in enrollment mix. How they will use the increased flexibility will depend in part on future changes in the competitive health care environment.

As indicated, health expenditures are typically lower for HMO enrollees than for persons covered by conventional insurance. A major issue is whether HMO enrollees also experience a slower rate of growth in costs. Data from several sources (Federal Employees Health Benefits Program, California State Employees, and Kaiser–Oregon) have been examined to compare trends in utilization and costs for HMO enrollees and comparison groups over periods of up to twenty-five years. Total costs can be broken down into cost per unit of service and the number of units, or utilization of services. Trends over time in cost per unit of service (for example, per hospital patient day) in HMOs are generally comparable to national cost trends, as are measures of factor inputs (such as office visits per physician per year). Trends in utilization, such as hospital days per one thousand enrollees, show slight reductions for HMO enrollees relative to persons with conventional coverage. Therefore, the rate of growth in total costs (including out-of-pocket expenses) is only slightly lower for persons in HMOs. While HMOs may offer lower costs at any point in time, they have not been able to substantially change the national patterns of medical care inflation and increasing resource use.[18]

Although the HMO enrollment trend has been upward, many persons have a sufficient level of dissatisfaction with HMOs to disenroll. Persons who disenrolled from a prepaid group practice, when compared with continuing members, have fewer health problems (as measured by bed disability and psychologic well-being), report access to HMOs difficult and inconvenient, and are less likely to have established a permanent relationship with a physician in the HMO plan. Enrollees who join the plan on the basis of more direct knowledge of its actual operation are more likely to continue in it.[19]

Health Maintenance Organizations and Competition

Discussions of HMO competition often assume that HMOs will attempt to maximize savings—that is, take maximum advantage of the various efficiencies inherent in the HMO structure; but prepaid plans may prefer, to borrow Herbert Simon's term, to "satisfice." If a plan is attempting to reach the break-even enrollment point or to grow rapidly, it does face incentives to offer relatively comprehensive benefits for the lowest possible price. This policy has high organizational costs, however, which any plan that is profitable and expanding rapidly will consider. One cost is that the strict utilization controls required to ensure that care is allocated efficiently and in accord with least-cost principles may alienate doctors and cause them to be in conflict with the administration of the HMO. Second, strict economies and efficiencies might give HMO enrollees the impression that the HMO provides poorer quality care than, for example, fee-for-service medical practitioners.

Goldberg and Greenberg argued that an increase in HMO market share would decrease Blue Cross hospitalization rates.[20] As HMOs attracted patients by means of lower premiums, broader benefits, or some other method, it was assumed that Blue Cross would attempt to keep its cost (and, therefore, premiums) comparable by implementing various hospital utilization controls. The authors analyzed 1974 state data on federal employees choosing the Blue Cross high option plan. The results were consistent with the hypothesis using both nonmaternity days per thousand and the average length of stay in maternity cases. However, the results are dominated by the activities in three West Coast states and Hawaii. When the four western states were omitted, the relationship between HMO share and Blue Cross utilization was no longer statistically significant.[21] This failure to incorporate the historically lower utilization of inpatient facilities on the West Coast potentially biased their results. Consequently their findings, though important, must be cautiously interpreted.

Some of the locations Goldberg and Greenberg studied are the sites of well-established and comparatively large HMOs. Washington, D.C., for example, is the location of the Group Health Association (GHA), a forty-year-old plan with roughly 110,000 members; and New York City is the home of the Health Insurance Plan of Greater New YorK (HIP), a thirty-year old plan with about 875,000 members. The Goldberg-Greenberg study indicates that the usual assumption that for any HMO to survive over time it must compete rigorously is too simplistic. Plans like GHA and HIP not only survive but apparently do not compete. This operating strategy may be perfectly appropriate for established plans which for reasons such as facility size or managerial philosophy are not eager to enroll more members. The managers may conclude that the probability of significant expansion is too low to justify the organizational costs required to maximize savings, minimize premiums, and at the same time provide comprehensive benefits.

These considerations have led some to argue that the benefits of competition and the positive effects of HMOs will only really occur when HMOs compete vigorously with each other. When this happens, it is maintained that efficiency will cause pressure for more efficiency. Recent experience in Minneapolis, where seven HMOs compete with one another, indicates that the effects of this competition are unclear.[22] Luft observed that despite a doubling of HMO enrollment in Minneapolis–St. Paul between 1975 and 1977, and

HMO hospital utilization averaging 42 percent below the Blue Cross group average, overall hospital use in the area remained constant or increased slightly, whereas the HMO reductions should have produced an overall decrease of fifteen days per one thousand even apart from a competitive effect. The result might be explained in a number of ways but is "consistent with both the notions of no major competitive response and selective enrollment of low utilizers in the HMOs."[23]

Thus, competition among HMOs may be expected to have its intended effects only if several conditions occur. First, the entrepreneurs and managers of HMOs must actually be willing to compete with each other. However, there is no obvious reason why this should be the case. Most HMO executives want their organizations to be successful rather than to test academic or scholarly concepts concerning competition. They succeed by establishing strong, stable organizations, not by attempting to woo individuals away from other HMOs. As one HMO administrator said, "Many HMOs would be happy with 25,000 subscribers, and having achieved this population to leave it right there. It's easier to manage."[24]

Second, in order for HMOs to compete with one another, employers must be willing to offer more than one HMO and perhaps also to encourage their employees to join a prepaid plan. To the extent that HMOs focus on one geographic area, this may be difficult. Employers are reluctant to bear the administrative costs of offering plans which are a great distance from the firm or near the homes of only a few workers. Some will offer a federally qualified HMO because they are legally required to do so (if and when one exists in their area), but will not offer any other HMO. Minneapolis appears to be a unique exception. Several major employers have not only encouraged their employees to join HMOs, but have vigorously promoted several HMOs simultaneously.

Third, the expectation of competition between HMOs assumes that unions will react positively to multiple HMOs and will leave the choice of particular plans to the individual union members. Unions sometimes welcome an HMO option as a bargaining point with conventional plans, the threat of taking their business elsewhere thus becoming real. Generally, however, unions prefer to commit their membership to maximize its influence by enrolling in one plan, not to fragment its influence among several.

Fourth, to be a feasible policy, competition among HMOs must ultimately be self-stabilizing. If aggressive HMOs greatly affect their competition, will the weak HMOs be allowed to shut down? Or, will the latter be allowed to continue, sacrificing efficiency in order to keep the ultimate consequence of competition from occurring?

This discussion implies that competition in health care should not be considered simply as an economic process, but also as the result of the interests of key people in formal organizations. The latter inlcudes HMO sponsors and managers, employers, unions, and those government agencies that regulate competition. The conditions required to support vigorous competition among HMOs are unlikely to be met for long periods in many places.

Medicare and HMOs

About 27 million people are eligible to receive services under the Medicare program, but only about 600,000 of those eligible (2.2 percent) were enrolled in HMOs or prepaid practice plans at the end of 1983.[25] Enrollment of eligibles in prepaid plans have been authorized since 1967 under Section 1833 of the Social Security Act. Enrollment gains have been steady and there has been a slightly faster rate of increase since 1972. However, most of the enrollment growth has been the result of "aging in," that is, people who are members of prepaid plans converting their membership when they become eligible for Medicare benefits.

In 1970, both Congress and the administration began to consider methods of containing the escalating costs of the Medicare program. Legislation was introduced in 1970 to permit the government to contract directly with HMOs and to provide prospective reimbursement at 95 percent of the prevailing Medicare fee-for-service costs. However, it was not until 1972 that agreement was reached to permit the government to contract with HMOs on either a cost or risk basis.

Congress, in a further effort to limit Medicare cost increases, amended the Social Security Act in 1976, adding Section 1876 which included specific conditions under which HMOs could contract to enroll Medicare beneficiaries on either a risk or cost basis. With a cost contract, the HMO is paid the "reasonable" costs of the covered services it furnishes to Medicare enrollees. With a risk-based contract, the total payment to the HMO is determined by comparing the HMO's adjusted per capita incurred cost of providing covered services to Medicare patients with the adjusted average per capita cost of providing such services to a similar beneficiary population outside the HMO. If the former cost is less than the latter, savings of up to 20 percent are shared equally by the HMO and the government. If the adjusted per capita incurred cost for treating Medicare patients is greater than the adjusted average per capita cost of treating the elderly population in general, the losses are borne by the HMO.[26]

These reimbursement mechanisms gave HMOs a choice between two alternative payment systems for Medicare enrollees. One was for the HMO to be paid on the basis of retrospectively determined costs. This required that the HMOs keep individual patient accounts and generate bills for services provided. This meant that HMOs acted essentially as if they were fee-for-service providers.[27]

The alternative payment scheme, by contrast, was consistent with the principles that govern the typical HMO operations. It provided for capitation payments to be made on behalf of Medicare enrollees, with payments determined on the basis of average health care costs for Medicare beneficiaries in the fee-for-service sector within the same location and adjusted for age, sex, and other factors. However, computation of the capitation rate, known as the adjusted average per capita cost (AAPCC) was criticized because it afforded HMOs little protection against adverse selection. Adverse selection could cause HMOs to lose money on Medicare enrollees since capitation revenues would be inadequate to cover the higher than average costs of severely ill elderly persons.

To calculate the AAPCC for an HMO, the Office of the Actuary of the Health Care Financing Administration (HCFA) first determined the overall per capita cost for all Medicare beneficiaries. The cost was multiplied by the age, sex, and geographic cost indexes that corresponded to the counties in which the HMO operated. The resulting figure represented Medicare's expected per capita cost for the beneficiaries in the HMO's service area. Finally, the service area per capita cost was adjusted to reflect the age, sex, welfare, and institutional status of beneficiary members of the particular HMO.[28]

Data used by HCFA to make these adjustments have been criticized as being outdated and wrong.[29] Moreover, it is generally agreed that the variables used to calculate and adjust the AAPCC were too few in number and that more factors must be included if the adjusted rate is to approximate with acceptable precision the expected cost of serving Medicare enrollees.[30] The single best adjusting factor for the AAPCC would likely be a measure of beneficiary health status,[31] an item not presently included.

Although the 1982 amendments to the Social Security Act specifically provided for inclusion of additional variables in determining the adjusted AAPCC, the likelihood that Medicare will incorporate a health status factor is small, since no generally acceptable method exists for directly measuring health status. In the absence of a capitation mechanism that adequately compensates for differences in individual's expected utilization, HMOs continued to be reluctant to enroll Medicare patients[32] because of the financial risks associated with adverse selection.

These incentives would change significantly, however, if a health status adjustment were to be incorporated into the AAPCC. The adjusting factor would reduce HMO concerns about the financial consequences of adverse selection. Because Medicare capitation would then approximate an experience-rated formula, a participating HMO "might even find high-risk people especially desirable because of the larger potential savings it could offer relative to the conventional system."[33]

Recent and Future HMO Developments

The widespread emphasis upon making health care delivery cost-effective may reduce the historic competitive advantage of HMOs. In particular, HMO administrators are well aware that their cost advantage has been mainly based upon their patients using hospitals less frequently than the patients of fee-for-service physicians. However, the diagnosis-related group (DRG) system gives hospitals the same incentive to reduce patients' length of stay, at least for Medicare patients, that HMOs have always had. Therefore, many hospitals are discharging Medicare patients as quickly as possible, which is reducing the length of stay for fee-for-service patients.

HMO administrators are concerned by the pressure to give their members access to expensive modern procedures such as heart and liver transplants. After advertising that members receive all the medical treatment they need, HMOs are embarrassed by unfavorable publicity when they are sued by their patients for refusing to pay for transplants. If HMOs are legally required to provide transplants, they fear they will become victims of adverse selection when people who think they may need a transplant decide to join.[34]

One important development affecting HMOs is the 1984 federal regulations which will encourage HMOs to enroll more Medicare patients. These regulations would permit HMOs to be paid 95 percent of what Medicare calculates it would have to pay in each area for fee-for-service care, the latter amount being adjusted for sex, age, welfare status, and other Medicare patient population variables. The Department of Health and Human Services (DHHS) estimates this care of Medicare patients will cost the government about $2,200 per patient annually, while the typical Medicare patient will have to pay $20 to $50 a month in additional premium charges. HMOs are expected to make a profit because it is believed that they can care for the average Medicare patient for less than 95 percent of the comparable cost under fee-for-service schemes, and they can retain the savings.

DHHS Secretary Margaret Heckler has estimated that over the next three to four years, HMOs could enroll another 600,000 Medicare beneficiaries who presently are served by other providers. However, she notes that in the initial period of this enrollment surge, the Medicare–HMO option will cost the government an additional $30 million per year.[35]

It is likely that future HMO development will be different from that of the past fifteen years. For example, rather than a continued proliferation of new HMOs, trends indicate that established ones will expand into other states or will affiliate with one another to form networks that will simplify employers' administrative work when more than one HMO is offered to employees. Also, hospitals and insurance companies are expected to own and manage more HMOs. In addition, a large number of HMOs will become for-profit companies rather than nonprofit organizations.

As HMOs grow, they will become more attractive for unions seeking to enroll their physicians. Many nurses employed in Kaiser HMOs are union members, and it is likely that HMO physician unions will become a reality in the near future. However, prospective organizers of HMO physician unions may have to deal with the phenomenon of a doctor surplus. Such a situation makes it easy not only for HMOs to hire physicians, but also to replace striking physicians or physicians who are union organizers.

HMOs have been a growing force on the American medical scene for most of the past fifty years. However, even with their recent rapid growth they enroll fewer than 8 percent of the American people and hire a somewhat smaller proportion of U.S. physicians. HMOs are not likely to disappear or to dominate American medicine. They will continue as one significant form of medical care delivery in an increasingly pluralistic medical system in which cost is playing an increasing role.

Preferred Provider Organizations

Preferred provider organizations (PPOs) are arrangements in which physicians, hospitals, or other providers contract to administer health care on a fee-for-service basis to set groups of beneficiaries. These contracts may be made with union trust funds, employers, insurance carriers, brokers, or other organizations.[36]

The essentials of a PPO include:

1. A panel of providers that agrees to establish fees which typically represent a discount from their usual charges.
2. There is no requirement that consumers limit themselves to those providers. However, consumer incentives in the form of reduced charges may be incorporated into the agreement.
3. Utilization review and data collection programs designed to help administrators assess the impact of a PPO on the cost and utilization of health benefits by employees.
4. Providers, in return for discounting services, receive rapid payment for patient care. Moreover, providers are sheltered from the risks of a closed-practice arrangement such as an HMO.
5. Employers have an opportunity to realize short-term savings from discounts, as well as long-term savings through constraints on utilization.

As PPOs evolve from primarily provider-based contracts with small employers and union trusts, to large-scale agreements with insurance companies and major corporations, practice arrangements are changing. For example, the most recently formed PPOs are no longer giving simple discounts, but instead are relying on strict utilization controls as a means of achieving cost savings. Such controls include preadmission screening and concurrent review of hospitalized patients, as well as retrospective claims review. Negotiated fee schedules and hospital reimbursement formulas based on established per diem rates or DRG charges are also replacing discounting.[37]

Physicians appear sharply divided between those who see PPOs as a means of guaranteeing a steady patient load and those who feel the price for that security is too high. Some physicians feel PPOs will bring about substantial reductions in future physician income levels and reduce quality of care. They fear a loss to outside concerns of the freedom to make critical decisions about the treatment of patients based on their best medical judgment.

Summary

Health maintenance organizations have grown steadily in number and membership in the 1970s and 1980s due to favorable legislation and rising premiums of conventional insurers. However, competition from hospitals and preferred provider organizations may slow the growth of enrollment in the future.

HMOs have had less impact on the health service industry than proponents originally expected. HMOs have achieved substantial cost savings for the participants, but most of this saving has been due to lower hospitalization rates as compared to groups with conventional insurance. Health costs of patients served by HMOs appear to increase at about the same rate as for persons not served by HMOs.

There is only limited evidence that HMOs compete with each other. It appears that once an HMO has achieved a reasonable size, its administrators put a greater emphasis on organizational stability than vigorous competition with other HMOs for enrollees.

Relatively few Medicare patients have traditionally joined HMOs. This was partly because the Medicare program provided little incentive for HMOs to enroll elderly patients. However, new policies established by the Department of Health and Human Services are expected to increase Medicare reimbursement to HMOs and provide incentives for the latter to enroll older persons.

Preferred provider organizations have been growing rapidly in the past five years. There is some indication that PPO practice arrangements are changing. There is less emphasis on price discounts and more reliance on utilization controls as a means of obtaining cost savings.

Notes

1. Gordon MacLeod and Jeffrey Prussin, "The Continuing Evolution of Health Maintenance Organizations," *New England Journal of Medicine* 288, no. 9 (March 1, 1973):440–41.

2. Clifton Gaus, Barbara Cooper, and Constance Hirschman, "Contrasts in HMO and Fee-for-Service Performance," *Social Security Bulletin* 39, no. 5 (May 1976):3.

3. Harold Luft, "Health Maintenance Organizations and the Rationing of Medical Care," *Milbank Memorial Fund Quarterly/Health and Society* 60, no. 2 (1982):271.

4. Gaus, Cooper, and Hirschman, op. cit., p. 4.

5. Samuel Meyers, "Growth in Health Maintenance Organizations," in *Health United States, 1981,* DHHS Publication (PHS) 82-1232 (Hyattsville, Md.: U.S. Department of Health and Human Services, 1981), p. 125.

6. J.M. Benyak, ed., *A Disgest of State Laws Affecting Prepayment of Medical Care Group Practice and HMOs* (Rockville, Md.: Health Law Center, Aspen Systems Corp., 1973), pp. 383–86.

7. Samuel Meyers, "Growth in Health Maintenance Organizations," in *Health United States, 1981,* DHHS Publication No. (PHS) 82-1232 (Hyattsville, Md.: U.S. Department of Health and Human Services, 1981) p. 134; "HMOs: A Decade of Growth," *Business Insurance,* December 19, 1983, p. 27; Harry Schwartz, "Competing for Dollars," *Private Practice* 16, no. 8 (August 1984):17, 19.

8. Harry Schwartz, "Competing for Dollars," *Private Practice* 16, no. 8 (August 1984):19.

9. Ibid., pp. 19–20.

10. See, for example, Harold S. Luft, "How Do Health Maintenance Organizations Achieve Their 'Savings'? Rhetoric and Evidence," *New England Journal of Medicine* 298, no. 24 (June 15, 1978):1336–43; Harold S. Luft, "HMOs and the Medical Care Market," in *Socioeconomic Issues of Health,* ed. Douglas Hough and Glen Misek, (Chicago: American Medical Association, Center for Health Services Research and Development, 1980), pp. 85–102; Frances Cunningham and John Williamson, "How Does the Quailty of Health Care in HMOs Compare to That in Other Settings? An Analytic Literature Review, 1958–79," *Group Health Journal* 1, no. 2 (Winter 1980):4–25; Frederic Wolensky, "The Performance of Health Maintenance Organizations: An Analytic Review," *Milbank Memorial Fund Quarterly/Health and Society* 57, no. 4 (Fall 1980):537–87.

11. Cunningham and Williamson, op. cit., pp. 4–25.

12. M.F. Collen, L.G. Dales, G.D. Fieldman, C.D. Flagle, R. Feldman, and A.B. Siegelaub, "Multiphasic Checkup Evaluation Study. Part 4. Preliminary Cost-Benefit Analysis for Middle-Aged Men," *Preventive Medicine* 2, no. 2 (1973):236–46.

13. D. Mechanic, *The Growth of Bureaucratic Medicine* (New York: Wiley-Interscience, 1976), p. 87.

14. Luft, "How Do Health Maintenance Organizations Achieve their 'Savings' " p. 1338.

15. G.B. Meier and J. Tellotson, *Physician Reimbursement and Hospital Use in HMOs* (Excelsior, Minn.: Interstudy, 1978), p. 19.

16. S.E. Berki and M.L.F. Ashcraft, "HMO Enrollment—Who Joins and Why: A Review of the Literature," *Milbank Memorial Fund Quarterly/Health and Society* 58, no. 4 (1980):588–632.

17. A.A. Scitovsky, L. Benham, and N. McCall, "Use of Physician Services Under Two Prepaid Plans," *Medical Care* 17, no. 5 (May 1979):441–60.

18. Harold Luft, "Trends in Medical Care Costs: Do HMOs Lower the Rate of Growth?" *Medical Care* 18, no. 1 (January 1980):1.

19. David Mechanic, Norma Weiss, and Paul Cleary, "The Growth of HMOs: Issues of Enrollment and Disenrollment," *Medical Care* 31, no. 3 (March 1983):338.

20. Lawrence Goldberg and Warren Greenberg, *The Health Maintenance Organization and Its Effects on Competition,* Staff Report to the Federal Trade Commission, July 1977 (Washington, D.C.), pp. 56–62.

21. Alain Enthoven, "Competition of Alternative Delivery Systems," in *Competition in the Health Care Sector,* ed. Warren Greenberg, (Germantown, Md.: Aspen Systems Corp., 1978), pp. 255–78.

22. J.B. Christianson and W. McClure, "Competition in the Delivery of Medical Care," *New England Journal of Medicine* 301, no. 15 (October 11, 1979), pp. 812–18.

23. H.S. Luft, "Health Maintenance Organizations, Competition, Cost Containment, and National Health Insurance," in *National Health Insurance, What Now, What Later, What Never?,* ed. Mark Pauly, (Washington, D.C.: American Enterprise Institute for Public Policy Research, 1980), p. 119.

24. Lawrence Brown, "Competition and Health Cost Containment: Cautions and Conjectures," *Milbank Memorial Fund Quarterly/Health and Society* 59, no. 2 (1981):168.

25. Daniel Waldo and Helen Lanzenby, "Demographic Characteristics and Health Care Use and Expenditures by the Aged in the United States: 1977–1984," *Health Care Financing Review* 6, no. 1 (Fall 1984), p. 15.

26. Myers, op. cit., p. 126.

27. J.W. Thomas, Richard Lichtenstein, Leon Wyszewianski, and S.E. Berki, "Increasing Medicare Enrollment in HMOs: The Need for Capitation Rates Adjusted for Health Status," *Inquiry* 20, no. 3 (Fall 1983):227–39.

28. P. Eggers, and R. Prihoda, "Pre-Enrollment Reimbursement Patterns of Medicare Beneficiaries Enrolled in 'At Risk' HMOs," *Health Care Financing Review* 4, no. 3 (September 1982):55–74.

29. S. Trieger, T.W. Galblum, and G. Riley, "HMOs: Issues and Alternatives for Medicare and Medicaid," *Health Care Financing Issues,* HCFA Publication No. 03107 (Washington, D.C.: Health Care Financing Administration, 1982), pp. 114–28.

30. Harold Luft, Judith Feder, John Holahan, and Karen D. Lennox, "Health Maintenance Organizations," in *National Health Insurance: Conflicting Goals and Policy Theories,* ed. Judith Feder, John Holahan, and Ted Marmor (Washington, D.C.: Urban Institute, 1980), pp. 129–80.

31. G. Anderson and J.R. Knidsman, "Patterns of Expenditures Among High Utilizers of Medical Care Services: The Experience of Medicare Beneficiaries from 1974 to 1977," paper presented at the annual meeting of the American Public Health Association, Montreal, Canada, November 1982.

32. T.W. Galbaum and S. Trieger, "Demonstrations of Alternative Delivery Systems Under Medicare and Medicaid," *Health Care Financing Review* 3, no. 3 (March 1982):1–12.

33. Harold Luft, "Health Maintenance Organizations and the Rationing of Medical Care," p. 282.

34. Schwartz, op. cit., p. 17.

35. Ibid., p. 19.

36. Suzanne Viau, *PPOs: The State of the Art* (Washington, D.C.: Health Care Publications, 1983), pp. 12–13.

37. Ibid., pp. 8, 13.

8
Recent Changes in the Delivery of Health Care

The health care delivery system in the United States is undergoing rapid change. Care in hospitals is to an increasing extent being replaced by treatment in less expensive facilities such as free-standing emergency centers or surgicenters. As consumers have become more knowledgeable regarding the importance of health care, self-treatment has become a more frequent source of care. While this has some advantages, particularly in regard to cost, there is also the possibility that some medical conditions will be unknown to patients and, therefore, untreated.

In response to the high costs of medical care, some patients are reducing their utilization of physician services. These individuals are relying more on nontraditional healers and health books which emphasize self-care. Some of these books are designed to help individuals undertake self-diagnosis and treatment without reliance on health professionals. Much of this literature is readily available to the general public. For example, a 1975 book, *How to be Your Own Doctor (Sometimes)*,[1] includes: a guide to self-care for common illnesses, injuries, and most emergencies; drug treatment; and symptom-concept and testing indices.[1] Lists identify brochures, guides, pamphlets, and other materials useful in building self-help concepts, knowledge, and skills.

The use of self-examination and self-care has been encouraged by some feminists who stress increased knowledge of anatomy and physiology, the risk of various sex-related illnesses, as well as techniques for self-examination. This view of health care behavior reflects to some extent the belief that the traditional male-dominated health care system has given inadequate attention to women's health care needs.

Over one million copies of *Take Care of Yourself: A Consumer's Guide to Medical Care* has been sold, mostly to insurance companies and local Blue Cross and Blue Shield organizations, who have distributed copies to their policy holders. The book has been so successful that a similar one was written about children's health for parents. Blue Cross and Blue Shield officials believe that if consumers follow these books' advice on various health problems and conditions, physician visits can be reduced.[2]

In addition to a large number of self-care health publications, a great variety of medical devices are presently being sold to consumers throughout the country. These include, in addition to such standard items as the thermometer, tests which indicate the amount of sugar in the urine, pregnancy test kits which cost about $10, and sphygmomanometers which measure blood pressure in arteries. Although tests to detect sugar in urine and blood pressure devices have long been available, the latter have only been marketed for home use during the past five years. With appropriate self-education, persons with hypertension can monitor their own blood pressure. Most doctors maintain that individuals should not view these devices as a complete substitute for physician care. However, the use of these home health aids may well reduce the number of physician visits.

Pregnancy test kits that give reliable results are fairly new. As with most laboratory tests, the results often indicate a few false negatives and a few false positives. When the results are negative, a pregnancy kit does substitute for a physician visit. However, in cases with positive test results, pregnancy kits seldom delay visits to a physician. Another recent health aid is self-care kits to detect breast cancer through heat-sensitive, specially prepared, paper-like strips that are placed on the breast.

A few physicians react positively to their patients' efforts at self-help, but most physicians oppose such activities. Some may feel uncomfortable if patients become aware of the basic uncertainties regarding diagnosis and treatment of many health conditions. Other physicians may find it easier to manage patients who have minimal health or medical knowledge since they are less likely to question the physician's treatment regimen.

Moreover, some physicians actively oppose self-care activities, particularly when information is provided under the auspices of nontraditional clinics. Self-help clinics are frequently operated by well-trained physicians and offer medically sound self-care techniques such as biofeedback, massage, and whirlpool baths to reduce stress. In addition, they teach people how to take one's own blood pressure, as well as how to interpret biochemical test results. While some doctors may honestly believe that the directors of holistic and wellness-oriented clinics are cultists or quacks, economists suspect that this opposition stems from the fact that these clinics attract patients who might otherwise seek traditional medical care and, thus, are in competition with more traditional health care providers.

There is considerable evidence that self-care programs can reduce health care costs. For example, organized self-care programs have proved cost-effective among those suffering chronic illnesses, which represents a growing proportion of total morbidity. For example, in a self-care program with hemophiliacs at the Tufts New England Medical Center, total cost per patient was lowered 45 percent in comparison with conventional treatment. A diabetic self-care program run by the University of Southern California reduced the number of patients experiencing diabetic coma by two-thirds, halved the number of emergency room visits, and saved hospitals and consumers $1.7 million over a two-year period.[3]

Home Health Care

Home health care is undergoing major changes. For years, home health care services have been widely considered in the context of the chronic care needs of the growing elderly population. From that standpoint, the term *home health care* usually refers to services that provide personnel to assist with activities ranging from bathing to various kinds of physical therapy. Their primary objective is to increase the patient's ability to cope with daily living.

Less widely known among the general population are the technology-based home health care services. These are increasingly available both to patients with certain chronic diseases and as a follow-up to acute care. This type of treatment includes home dialysis, cancer chemotherapy, and inhalation therapy using the new oxygen concentrators. This technology-based home health care is more aggressive than the traditional personal services kind of care. It is considered a mechanism for reducing utilization of relatively costly hospital services. The charges for these home treatments tend to be below inpatient charges because only the cost of the staff and the materials specifically applicable to the therapy are included in total costs.

In general, home health care is frequently more comfortable and less anxiety-producing for the patient and more convenient to the family than institutional care. However, until recently, home health care was less adequately covered by insurance than, for example, hospital care. The extent of coverage of home health care by third-party payers is beginning to improve. Physicians generally support an expansion of home health care because these services can reduce the cost to the patient without causing the doctor to lose control over the treatment regimen.

New Childbirth Alternatives

No longer is the traditional maternity ward the only institutional set-up for childbirth. Free-standing birthing centers and homelike alternative birth centers within hospitals are growing in popularity.

Birthing Centers

Birthing centers are the most recent development in regard to free-standing treatment centers. Although these centers have been in operation in Europe for many years, the first in America began operation in 1975, sponsored by the Maternity Center Association in New York City. The country now has more than 100 free-standing birthing centers providing women with an alternative to traditional hospital or home delivery. Women generally are admitted when they are in the final stages of labor. A typical stay is four to six hours, after which the mother and baby go home.[4] In a sense, these centers are an updated version of the maternity hospitals that were commonplace before World War I.

The growth of birthing centers has been opposed by the American College of Obstetricians and Gynecologists (ACOG), which believes that hospitals provide the safest place for delivery for both mother and child. They also prefer that birthing centers be located within hospital settings because safeguards can be provided in the case of an unexpected difficult delivery. Between 10 and 30 percent of high-risk situations occur among low-risk mothers. These high-risk patients cannot be screened for hospital delivery in advance.[5] Birthing centers need appropriate physician and hospital affiliation to handle unexpected occurrences.

However, nearly half the birthing centers presently in existence are owned and operated by physicians who do comply with ACOG standards. Most of the remainder are operated by nurse–midwives or groups of women who have established the centers because of a perceived need in a particular location.

A growing number of women are delivering their children in birth centers. This is a positive development for the health insurance industry because birth centers can reduce the cost of a delivery by as much as 50 percent. The average hospital charge for a normal birth is $1,713. A 1982 National Association of Birthing Centers (NABC) survey found the average birth center charge is $801.[6]

Many insurers now include reimbursement of approved birth centers as a regular part of their medical coverage. In fact, many insurers are willing to pay the total cost for birth center deliveries without charging hospital patients the usual deductibles. Thus, Blue Cross/Blue Shield of New Hampshire even offers mothers a $50 cash rebate for delivering babies in birth centers. This insurer also provides nursing and homemaker benefits.

Although they accept as patients only mothers with low-risk childbirths, birthing centers are obtaining a small but growing share of maternity cases. Between 1975 and 1980, the National Center for Health Statistics estimates the number of children delivered each year outside of hospitals increased 30 percent to more than 35,000,[7] with about 10,000 deliveries a year occurring in free-standing birth centers.

Hospitals have responded to the competition associated with out-of-hospital delivery by transforming unused labor rooms into more home-like birthing rooms. Besides giving a variety of gifts to the new mother, some hospitals offer maternity fashion shows and free health club memberships to mothers who want to get back in shape after delivery.

The National Association of Birthing Centers says that about a dozen states have adopted regulations for birthing center staffs and services. At least seventeen more are drafting regulations providing for licensing of personnel and establishment of safety standards.

Local physicians' attitudes are important regarding the success of a birth center. Their opposition can even prevent one from opening. For example, Capital Health Care recently abandoned plans for a birth center in Salem, Oregon. Doctors there were unwilling to permit midwives to deliver babies and worried about the length of time of deliveries, since birthing centers are reluctant to hasten labor with drugs.

The growing surplus of physicians (see chapter 3 for a discussion of this surplus) and the fact that birthing centers are proliferating, may soften opposition among physicians. Moreover, an increasing number of physicians are interested either in joint ventures with entrepreneurs or in establishing centers themselves. They want to protect their market and they are responding to insurers' concern about rising medical costs.

Some patients find birthing centers unsatisfactory. These mothers complain about the fact that they returned home in only twenty-four hours when they would have preferred a longer stay.

The experience of an alternative birth center in Jacksonville, Florida, is fairly typical. One hundred eleven patients were accepted into the center during the two-year period from April 1980 to April 1982. Of these twenty-two were transferred antepartum, eighteen were transferred intrapartum, and seventy-one labored and delivered at the center. There were no fetal or maternal losses during this period.

The only maternal complication occurring among the seventy-one patients delivering at the center was one case of postpartum atony which did not require blood transfusion or maternal transfer, and eventually responded to oxytocics. There were no other incidents of maternal or fetal morbidity.

The overall caesarean section rate for these seventy-one patients who labored at the alternative birthing center was 34 percent and the total cost of $950 (as compared with over $2,000 for a physician-assisted hospital birth) was typical of free-standing birth centers.[8]

Hospital Alternative Birth Centers (ABCs)

Hospital alternative birth centers generally consist of one or two postpartum rooms where an attempt is made to create a homelike atmosphere for the hospital birth. Some hospital ABCs have furnishings such as a dresser, queen-sized bed, carpeting, hanging plants, pictures, a stereo, overstuffed chairs, and a dining table.[9] In order to determine which mothers are permitted to labor and deliver in this setting, hospital committees have developed written protocols listing criteria for admission to the ABC and events necessitating transfer to the regular labor and delivery unit from the ABC.

Assuming that they conform to these protocols, throughout normal laboring, paturient, and early postpartum, women can give birth in an ABC with a minimum of routine medical procedures. The newborn's family and friends are free to interact without the traditional interference and separation imposed by the institution. Some ABCs provide for discharge home in six to twelve hours after birth, with postpartum follow-up home visits by center personnel.

Data from the states of Washington and California indicate the popularity of the ABCs. In 1979, more than 60 percent of all hospitals with obstetric services in Washington either had or planned to have alternative birth rooms. In California the number of ABCs increased from just three in 1975 to more than 120 in 1982. Recent data indicate that physicians and hospital administrators might be realizing their goal of bringing some of the home-birth population into the ABC. After a steady five-year increase, the percentage of out-of-hospital births declined in 1978 and 1979.[10]

However, uncooperative physicians, minimal demand by consumers, and overly strict hospital protocols are all factors associated with the limited use of hospital ABCs in the country as a whole. A number of obstetricians will not attend mothers in an alternative birth center or will attempt to persuade them not to use the facility.

Hospital alternative birth centers have attracted only 2.5 percent to 15 percent of expectant mothers even though at least 60 percent of these patients can be treated safely in the hospital ABC.[11] The hospital ABC, as it presently exists, may best be regarded as an attempt not only to compete with the alternative childbirth movement, but to retain medical control in order to continue the routine obstetrical procedures and interventions traditionally associated with normal childbirth.

Emergency Centers

In many areas of the country, hospitals and clinics are facing stiff competition from free-standing treatment centers. These centers are praised by some as a welcome return to more convenient medical care that was traditionally associated with physician housecalls. Others categorize them as "fast-food medicine," "store-front medicine," or "doc-in-the-box."[12]

Free-standing emergency care centers provide episodic emergency care twenty-four hours a day, seven days a week. Designed to serve critically ill patients who arrive by ambulance, they differ little from hospital emergency rooms, except that they are free-standing or independent of hospitals. They must, however, have a close working relationship with an inpatient facility in order to appropriately treat or refer serious cases.

Urgent care centers are a more recent development. These centers provide, at a minimum, episodic care for routine or minor emergency problems such as sore throats, sprains, lacerations, and simple fractures. Many of these centers are also beginning to provide continuing care. They are generally open twelve to sixteen hours a day, seven days a week. They specifically do not receive patients brought by ambulance since they do not have the facilities to handle seriously ill patients. They do provide some laboratory and radiology services. These centers are staffed by physicians and a small number of support personnel. Each nonphysician employee is usually given more than one task in order to increase the center's overall efficiency.

According to a 1983 survey by the National Association of Free-standing Emergency Centers (NAFEC), physicians owned 72.9 percent of FECs.[13] However, ownership trends are changing. Hospitals and universities are establishing some satellite centers. In addition, large corporations are beginning to develop the centers as a form of diversification in the health care field. Among the most widely known examples are Humana's Med First Operations and Charter Medical's Immediate Care Centers.

Both of these corporate examples appear to be hybrid organizations since they provide urgent as well as primary care. Such institutions may become more common in the future since an increasing number of hospital systems and individual hospitals are seeking ways to attract patients away from physician's offices. However, while these centers are frequently more accessible than a particular physician, their charges tend to be more than a physician's fee for an office visit.

A study by Burns found that about half of the centers had an annual budget of from $240,000 to $480,000. The budgets of 37 percent ranged from $500,000 to $2 million, and those of 11 percent of the centers ranged from $60,000 to $144,000 annually. A full 92 percent of the hospital-associated free-standing emergency centers share overhead with their parent institutions.[14]

In the decade since emergency and urgent care centers first developed, fees have been kept stable through cost-cutting techniques that have placed pressure on private physicians and hospital emergency rooms. Center development costs range from $250,000 to $500,000. A clinic with sixty patients a day can gross $800,000 to $900,000 a year.

According to the National Association for Ambulatory Care, treatment of a cut requiring stitches costs $133 at a hospital emergency room and $75 at an urgent care center. Treatment of an upper respiratory infection is $136 at an emergency room and $34 at an urgent care clinic.[15]

Free-standing emergency centers receive most of their revenues from private insurers. They receive somewhat less from self-paying patients, and a very small amount from Medicare and Medicaid. Twenty-one percent of the facilities reported that their entire source of funds were from self-paying patients. These emergency centers bill the patients directly, and the patient is reimbursed by a third-party payer.[16]

Estimates of the size of the potential market range between $2 billion and $5 billion per year.[17] The number of FECs is expected to reach 2,500 by mid-1985, according to the NAFEC.[18] However, the total size of the market ultimately depends on two factors: the success these institutions have in attracting emergency room patients, and the degree to which they can attract patients who presently utilize physicians' offices.

Unlike such competitive forces as preferred provider organizations which aim primarily for business from major insurers, free-standing treatment centers focus their marketing efforts directly on individual patients. Emergency clinics or urgent care centers are open considerably more hours than the typical physician's office and have lower patient charges than the usual hospital emergency department. One reason for the growth of these centers is the public's frustration at not being able to reach personal physicians on short notice. Moreover, given the mobility of our society, many people do not have a personal physician because they are recent arrivals in an area.

Contracts, joint ventures, and acquisitions between free-standing emergency centers and health maintenance organizations are increasing. Alternative health care providers are finding it more difficult to survive outside a network. For alternative health care providers, networking means that patients can receive more comprehensive, and often less expensive, care. However, for hospitals who own a relatively small number of FECs, it may mean a further reduction of utilization, especially when networking results in patients utilizing nonhospital facilities.

HMOs are contracting with FECs to provide health care services to HMO members during hours when the HMO is closed. The HMO obtains the benefit of decentralization and additional convenience for its members, as well as an alternative to more expensive emergency department referrals for weekend and evening hours. The HMO also retains greater control over patient flows and referrals. The FEC receives additional revenues and a guaranteed cash flow when the contract provides for capitation payments. Cooperation between HMOs and FECs results in decreasing traditional hospital emergency room use. However, without a contract, HMO patients who go to FECs during hours when the HMOs are not open often experience considerable delay in being reimbursed. FECs are established to provide the maximum possible convenience to patients, whereas HMOs establish some limits on convenience in order to reduce utilization.

Licensure and Regulation

FECs may be either hospital satellite clinics or nonaffiliated, for-profit corporations owned by groups of doctors or other investors. In many states the law perceives them as physicians' offices which subjects them to less regulation and which makes them less expensive and easier to operate than hospital departments offering similar services.

However, there is a general consensus that accreditation and/or licensure of free-standing emergency facilities will occur in the near future. One major reason for accreditation of health care facilities is the protection of the public from abuse. Another reason is to reduce the number of facilities providing services.

One appropriate control mechanism for the growing number of emergi-centers is licensure, and much of the impetus for licensure will probably come from third-party payers. Indeed these institutions may require that an emergi-center be licensed before it can receive reimbursement as an emergency department rather than as a physician's office.[19]

Emergency Centers as Competition for Hospital Emergency Departments

The growth of emergency centers raises the question of whether they reduce the number of hospital emergency department outpatient visits. In fact, emergency department visits to hospitals in the service areas of free-standing emergency centers have continued to grow. This strongly suggests that the presence of FECs has not led to a decline in emergency department visits to hospitals in their service areas. However, one cannot say whether FECs have reduced the rate of growth of emergency department visits to such hospitals.[20]

Because FECs are a relatively new alternative for health care provision, some people have supposed that health care consumers might substitute FECs for hospital emergency visits as a source of health care. However, FECs generally are designed to provide a convenient source of care to patients with non-life-threatening problems. As such, they may not be perceived by consumers as a replacement for hospital emergency departments, but instead, as a substitute for private physicians' offices. Thus, the presence of FECs in an area may affect the annual volume of visits to physicians' offices rather than visits to outpatient departments.

It is also possible that some consumers who visited an FEC would not otherwise have sought any professional medical attention. They may have believed that their problems were not sufficiently serious to warrant a hospital visit, and may not have had a regular source of care. In the absence of an FEC their medical problems might have gone untreated.

Other alternatives to the hospital emergency department may be masking a potential effect of FECs on emergency visits. FECs were developed because it was recognized that there was an unmet demand for unscheduled care. Walk-in clinics sponsored by HMOs and hospitals are increasingly available. Thus, hospitals that are outside the service area of FECs may be inside the service area of one of these other health care alternatives. Like hospitals with FECs nearby, these hospitals may lose potential emergency patients to the other health provider alternatives.[21]

Ambulatory Surgery Centers

In the early 1970s, free-standing ambulatory surgery centers were established. The first unit began operating in Phoenix, Arizona, and by early 1981 had performed over 70,000 surgical procedures with no deaths and no emergency hospital transfers. These centers are independent of hospitals and usually provide a full range of services for the types of surgery that can be performed on an outpatient basis. Community surgeons are granted operating privileges and can perform surgery in these facilities whenever the patient agrees and it is considered medically appropriate. Outpatient surgical procedures are performed on a scheduled basis in these centers. It is estimated that about 50 percent of all surgery can be performed in outpatient settings at present and that percentage may be increasing.

By 1982 there were approximately 100 to 150 free-standing surgical centers in the United States. The number of centers is growing rapidly with at least fifty new centers each year.

Most free-standing surgery centers are presently owned by groups of doctors, but medical corporations are also beginning to establish centers. The centers generally have no permanent staff of surgeons but gain revenues from fees charged to area surgeons who use the facilities to perform minor surgery.

When free-standing surgery centers first began developing, they were strongly opposed by hospital administrators who were concened about the competition for patients. However, hospitals have now recognized the need for ambulatory surgery and opposition has diminished.

Ambulatory Surgery Centers and Technological Change

The growth of ambulatory surgery occurred concomitantly with major advances in anesthesia. There are now types of anesthesia that can keep patients asleep between thirty minutes and twelve hours and yet those patients can return home shortly after awakening.[22] It is doubtful that cost-saving ambulatory surgery could have expanded rapidly if open-drop ether was still generally used since with the latter the anesthesiologist could not precisely control the anesthesia. Moreover, after awakening, the patient was generally groggy for a considerable period of time. Thus, the growth of free-standing surgery centers was greatly dependent on improved anesthetics.

Another technological change that fostered the growth of ambulatory surgery was diagnostic imaging. As technology has evolved from plain-film radiography to CT scanners, and now to nuclear magnetic resonance, the exploration of free-standing imaging clinics has intensified. More generally, this process has reduced the use of invasive diagnostic techniques.

As an increasing amount of work is done noninvasively, physicians are removing more and more diagnostic testing from hospitals to free-standing units. Instead of having the hospital's emphasis on treatment, these centers are specifically designed to meet the needs of diagnosticians. Work done in this environment is also less costly to the patient. Hence, changing economic incentives coupled with scientific developments are resulting in a shift in the patterns of medical diagnosis.

Cost Containment

A recent study by Blue Cross concluded that ambulatory surgery is the most important tool now available for slowing the rise in health care costs. Blue Shield of California has a list of more than 700 surgical procedures it recommends be done on an outpatient basis. Medicare has specified 100 procedures for which outpatient surgery is appropriate and for which hospitalization costs will not normally be reimbursed. Medi-Cal, the medical assistance program for low-income residents of California, has a similar list of 282 procedures.[23]

Hospital-Based Ambulatory Surgery Centers

Some hospitals are establishing or expanding ambulatory services because of increased competition from other providers of such services. However, in general, competition in the hospital industry has traditionally not been based on price differentials. Instead, hospitals have competed with each other in terms of the quality of care provided. This is a function of the level of technology used in patient care and the qualifications of the attending medical staff. Thus, physicians would hospitalize their patients in the facilities that they believed would lead to the best treatment outcomes.

In ambulatory surgery, there is selective competition among hospitals and independent groups of physicians. Ambulatory care providers seek patients who are able to pay for services. There may be price competition because the population has less insurance coverage for ambulatory services than it does for inpatient care. Because patients may pay more of the costs of ambulatory care themselves, they will be more sensitive to charges. Thus, providers are likely to set their charges at prevailing community levels to remain price-competitive.

A hospital that is not making full use of resources for inpatient care might be uninterested in an ambulatory surgery program because that would reduce its revenues from inpatient stays and increased excess bed capacity.[24] However, if a competitor, such as another hospital or private physician group, established an ambulatory surgery clinic, the hospital might be prompted to establish one in order to maintain its competitive position.

A recent American Hospital Association study found that 70 percent of hospitals surveyed offer ambulatory surgery and 87 percent use their main surgical suites for both inpatient and ambulatory surgery. The survey indicated that an average of 18 percent of all surgical procedures performed are done on an ambulatory basis.[25]

A prospective study of 13,433 patients at a free-standing ambulatory surgical center was performed. Virtually all of the patients were followed up through the first two postoperative weeks. One hundred six medical, surgical, or anesthetic complications were identified in the patient population. No deaths occurred in the center, and there was no instance of cardiovascular collapse. Sixteen patients were transferred to a general hospital. This study shows that many surgical procedures can be performed as safely in surgicenters as in the traditional hospital inpatient setting.[26]

Infection in Ambulatory Surgery

The remarkably low incidence of infection associated with ambulatory surgery is one of the major benefits of this procedure. Nearly one-fifth of infants admitted to the hospital for hernia surgery may obtain upper respiratory or gastrointestinal tract infections. The incidence of these infections was reduced 50 to 70 percent when the surgery was performed on an outpatient basis.

The reduction in postoperative infections associated with ambulatory surgery has also been observed in a population of elderly patients.[27] Williamson has performed almost three thousand cataract procedures in the outpatient setting and has stated that the ambulatory patient has less chance of experiencing pneumonia, cross-infection, and pulmonary embolism than those who become hospital inpatients.[28]

The reduction in the rate of infection requires adherence to accepted standards of sterile technique and common sense. However, it does not require the utilization of sophisticated techniques or costly equipment.

Cost Savings in Surgicenters—Two Case Studies

Patients who use ambulatory surgery instead of inpatient elective surgery can avoid from one to three days of hospitalization and associated daily charges for services such as radiology and pharmacy.[29]

A Phoenix free-standing pediatric surgicenter had a major impact on health care costs. The surgicenter charge for the two hundred fifty herniorraphies performed was $140 each. This cost included the use of the operating and recovery rooms, all medications and supplies, and all laboratory work done in the facility. It did not include professional fees (surgery, anesthesia, and pathology) that were billed privately by the providers. Admission to a hospital in Phoenix for the same operation would have meant two days of hospitalization and would have cost a minimum of $235. There was, therefore, an average saving of $95 per case, or a total saving of approximately $23,750 for the entire group.[30]

Cost analysis of all types of cases now being handled in the surgicenter, both adult and pediatric, has revealed an average reduction in billed charges of $135 per case as compared to charges for the same procedures performed in other Phoenix hospitals.[31] These savings are possible because the surgicenter is a maximum efficiency and special service facility, and the patient pays only his direct costs. There is no cross-subsidization of other hospital services.

Crouse–Irving Memorial Hospital's surgery center has been in operation since November 1976. It is located across the street from the hospital. The cost of having any specific procedure performed in the surgery center is about 20 percent of the cost of having the same procedure performed in the hospital. Total savings from 1976 to 1980 have been $10 million.[32]

Given the volume that the surgery center has been handling, one issue of concern has been utilization of the hospital. From 1976 to 1979, the number of beds in service remained constant at 536, while admissions and discharges decreased; however, the average daily census increased from 432 to 476; the occupancy rate increased from 82 percent to 89 percent, and the average length of stay increased from 6.3 days to 7.2 days.

Average weekend census rose from 395 in 1976 to 453 in 1979. The major reason for this increase was that most major-surgery patients required longer recuperation periods.

In effect, the surgery center has resulted in the hospital becoming, to a considerable degree, an intensive care facility. In addition to accommodating more major-surgery patients, the hospital also now has more beds available for other critically ill persons.

Since no other hospital in the state has a similar surgery center (with the resulting emphasis on more intensive care in the hospital), reimbursement has presented difficulties. Third-party rates are computed through comparison with hospitals not having surgery centers, thereby penalizing Crouse–Irving. However, some of the difference in revenue is made up by the increased census and longer length of stay.[33] The surgery center is a major cost containment unit because it removes from the facility the burden of sharing certain costs that are inherent in only the hospital's operation.

Advantages and Disadvantages

A major criticism of all free-standing treatment centers is that they are only able to care for patients with relatively minor medical problems, which increases the severity caseload for hospitals. Many hospital administrators are concerned that reducing the number of hospital patients needing low-cost services will tend to raise the costs of more serious care. Proponents of free-standing centers, however, maintain that center growth could actually reduce hospital costs in the long run, as hospitals would be able to eliminate services they no longer need to provide.

The growth of free-standing treatment centers offers new opportunities for the young physician in a field where a manpower surplus is becoming more common. (See chapter 3.) A physician employed in a free-standing center can practice without incurring the debts that occur when one buys into or purchases a practice. Moreover, as medicine becomes increasingly specialized, the centers could provide opportunities for specialists who wish to allocate some of their time to delivering primary health care services.

If the need for additional ambulatory surgical capacity exists, free-standing facilities are preferable. However, if the surgical capacity in a community is excessive, hospital-based ambulatory surgery programs are preferable. The marginal costs incurred could be minimal, and the savings to the community could be greater than those achieved by free-standing facilities, which would have to be constructed.

Summary

The rapid growth in health care costs has stimulated numerous changes in the health care delivery system and in consumer attitudes toward the health care system in general.

The self-care movement is an attempt by consumers to treat a variety of health care problems without resort to physician or clinic services. While this may save the consumer money, the key question from the standpoint of health care is how frequently consumers misdiagnose their own ailments and what are the consequences of misdiagnosis in regards to, for example, the delay in obtaining treatment from a health care provider.

While alternative birth centers are increasing in popularity, a very small proportion of mothers deliver in these facilities. These centers are primarily owned and operated by physicians and midwives. The cost of a delivery in a free-standing birth center is approximately one-half the cost of hospital delivery. While birth centers are a viable alternative for normal deliveries, between 10 percent and 30 percent of high-risk situations are associated with low-risk mothers, who cannot at present be screened for hospital delivery prior to the actual birth.

Emergency care centers and urgent care centers provide substitutes for emergency room and physician's office visits. Institutions offering both emergency and primary care are likely to become more common in the near future.

Free-standing emergency centers and HMOs are joining forces to provide health care networks providing comprehensive care at relatively low cost. The HMO obtains an alternative to more expensive emergency department referrals when the HMO is not open.

It is likely that free-standing emergency centers will be licensed or accredited in the future. The major impetus for regulation will likely be third-party payers.

Free-standing ambulatory surgery centers have grown rapidly since the late 1960s. The growth of these centers has been stimulated by a desire to hold down surgical costs and by technological change in the provision of anesthesia. Moreover, as noninvasive diagnostic techniques have become more common, it has become increasingly feasible to provide these services in surgicenters.

Research indicates that surgery can often be performed as safely in free-standing surgicenters as in hospitals. Moreover, in many cases the rate of infection among patients treated in surgicenters is lower than that among hospital inpatients.

One criticism of all free-standing treatment centers is that they skim off the less severe cases. Thus, the severity level of the typical hospital patient may tend to increase.

Notes

1. Lowell S. Levin, Alfred Katz, and Rick Holst, *Self-Care: Lay Initiatives in Health* (New York: Prodest, 1976), p. 108.

2. Rita Ricardo-Campbell, *The Economics and Politics of Health* (Chapel Hill: The University of North Carolina Press, 1982), p. 71.

3. Bruce Stokes, "Self-Care: A Nation's Best Health Insurance," *Science* 205, no. 4406 (August 10, 1979):547.

4. Cheryl Katz, "Free-standing Treatment Centers: Another Member of the Competition," *Postgraduate Medicine* 74, no. 2 (August 1983):294.

5. J.R. Brandstrader, "As More Women Have Babies in Birth Centers, Hospitals Re-think Obstetric Procedures," *Wall Street Journal*, November 29, 1983, p. 60.

6. Ibid.

7. Ibid.

8. Edward Zabrek, Patricia Simon, and Guy Benrubi, "The Alternative Birth Center in Jacksonville, Florida: The First Two Years," *Journal of Nurse–Midwifery* 28, no. 4 (July–August 1983):31.

9. Raymond DeVries, "Image and Reality: An Evaluation of Hospital Alternative Birth Centers," *Journal of Nurse–Midwifery* 28, no. 3 (May–June 1983):4.

10. Ibid., p. 4.

11. Ibid., p. 8.

12. Katz, op. cit., p. 291.

13. Jo Ellen Mistarz, "Hospitals Contracting with FECs," *Hospitals*, July 1, 1984, p. 36.

14. Linda Burns and Mindy Ferber, "Free-standing Emergency Care Centers Create Public Policy Issues," *Hospitals*, May 16, 1981, p. 74.

15. Suzanne Harper, "Clinics Add Convenience to Health Care," *USA Today*, February 26, 1985, p. 2-A.

16. Linda Burns and Mindy Ferber, op. cit., p. 74.

17. John Morley, III and Penelope Roeder, "New Opportunities for Out-of-Hospital Health Services," *New England Journal of Medicine* 310, no. 3 (January 19, 1984):195.

18. Mistarz, op. cit., p. 41.

19. Jerome Koncen, "Experts Examine Major Issues Facing Emergicenters," *Hospitals*, May 16, 1981, p. 90.

20. Mindy Ferber, "Impact of Free-standing Emergency Centers on Hospital Emergency Department Use," *Annals of Emergency Medicine* 12, no. 7 (1983):432.

21. Ibid.

22. Morley and Roeder, op. cit., p. 195.

23. Katz, op. cit., p. 293.

24. Linda Burns, "Ambulatory Surgery Growing at a Rapid Pace," *AORN Journal* 35, no. 2 (February 1982):268.

25. Ibid.

26. Herbert Natof, "Complications Associated with Ambulatory Surgery," *Journal of the American Medical Association* 244, no. 10 (September 5, 1980):1116.

27. Natof, op. cit., p. 1118.

28. D.E. Williamson, "The Cataract Patient: The Postoperative Regimen," in R.J. Brockhurst et al., eds., *Controversy in Ophthalmology* (Philadelphia: W.B. Saunders Co., 1977), pp. 125–36.

29. Randolph Grossman, "Is Ambulatory Surgery Less Expensive?" *Hospitals*, May 16, 1979, p. 112.

30. Daniel Cloud, Wallace Reed, John Ford, Laurence Linkner, David Trump, and George Dorman, "The Surgicenter: A Fresh Concept in Outpatient Pediatric Surgery," *Journal of Pediatric Surgery* 7, no. 2 (April 1972):211.

31. Ibid.

32. James Maher, "Unit Improves Surgical Costs and Utilization," *Hospitals*, September 16, 1980, p. 110.

33. Ibid.

Index

About the Author

Alan L. Sorkin is professor and chairman of the Department of Economics at the University of Maryland, Baltimore County. He also holds appointments in the Department of Epidemiology and Social Medicine of the University of Maryland Medical School and the Department of International Health of The Johns Hopkins University School of Hygiene and Public Health. He received his Ph.D. in economics from Johns Hopkins in 1966. Dr. Sorkin is the author of *American Indians and Federal Aid* (The Brookings Institution, 1971) and the following volumes published by Lexington Books: *Education, Unemployment, and Economic Growth* (1974), *Health Economics: An Introduction* (1975; revised second edition, 1984), *Health Economics in Developing Countries* (1976), *Health Manpower: An Economic Perspective* (1977), *The Urban American Indian* (1978), *The Economics of the Postal System* (1980), and *Economic Aspects of Natural Hazards* (1982). He has also written a number of articles focusing on the economics of human resources.